# GULF WAR and HEALTH
## Long-Term Effects of
## Blast Exposures

Committee on Gulf War and Health:
Long-Term Effects of Blast Exposures

Board on the Health of Select Populations

INSTITUTE OF MEDICINE
*OF THE NATIONAL ACADEMIES*

THE NATIONAL ACADEMIES PRESS
Washington, D.C.
**www.nap.edu**

**THE NATIONAL ACADEMIES PRESS**     500 Fifth Street, NW     Washington, DC 20001

NOTICE: The project that is the subject of this report was approved by the Governing Board of the National Research Council, whose members are drawn from the councils of the National Academy of Sciences, the National Academy of Engineering, and the Institute of Medicine. The members of the committee responsible for the report were chosen for their special competences and with regard for appropriate balance.

This study was supported by Contract VA241-P-2024 between the National Academy of Sciences and the Department of Veterans Affairs. Any opinions, findings, conclusions, or recommendations expressed in this publication are those of the authors and do not necessarily reflect the view of the organizations or agencies that provided support for this project.

International Standard Book Number-13:  978-0-309-26764-9
International Standard Book Number-10:  0-309-26764-1

Additional copies of this report are available from the National Academies Press, 500 Fifth Street, NW, Keck 360, Washington, DC 20001; (800) 624-6242 or (202) 334-3313; http://www.nap.edu.

For more information about the Institute of Medicine, visit the home page at: **www.iom.edu**.

The serpent has been a symbol of long life, healing, and knowledge among almost all cultures and religions since the beginning of recorded history. The serpent adopted as a logotype by the Institute of Medicine is a relief carving from ancient Greece, now held by the Staatliche Museen in Berlin.

Suggested citation: IOM (Institute of Medicine). 2014. *Gulf War and health, volume 9: Long-term effects of blast exposures*. Washington, DC: National Academies Press.

*"Knowing is not enough; we must apply.
Willing is not enough; we must do."*
—Goethe

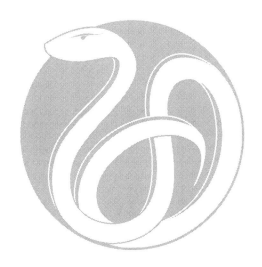

# INSTITUTE OF MEDICINE
*OF THE NATIONAL ACADEMIES*

**Advising the Nation. Improving Health.**

# THE NATIONAL ACADEMIES
## Advisers to the Nation on Science, Engineering, and Medicine

The **National Academy of Sciences** is a private, nonprofit, self-perpetuating society of distinguished scholars engaged in scientific and engineering research, dedicated to the furtherance of science and technology and to their use for the general welfare. Upon the authority of the charter granted to it by the Congress in 1863, the Academy has a mandate that requires it to advise the federal government on scientific and technical matters. Dr. Ralph J. Cicerone is president of the National Academy of Sciences.

The **National Academy of Engineering** was established in 1964, under the charter of the National Academy of Sciences, as a parallel organization of outstanding engineers. It is autonomous in its administration and in the selection of its members, sharing with the National Academy of Sciences the responsibility for advising the federal government. The National Academy of Engineering also sponsors engineering programs aimed at meeting national needs, encourages education and research, and recognizes the superior achievements of engineers. Dr. C. D. Mote, Jr., is president of the National Academy of Engineering.

The **Institute of Medicine** was established in 1970 by the National Academy of Sciences to secure the services of eminent members of appropriate professions in the examination of policy matters pertaining to the health of the public. The Institute acts under the responsibility given to the National Academy of Sciences by its congressional charter to be an adviser to the federal government and, upon its own initiative, to identify issues of medical care, research, and education. Dr. Harvey V. Fineberg is president of the Institute of Medicine.

The **National Research Council** was organized by the National Academy of Sciences in 1916 to associate the broad community of science and technology with the Academy's purposes of furthering knowledge and advising the federal government. Functioning in accordance with general policies determined by the Academy, the Council has become the principal operating agency of both the National Academy of Sciences and the National Academy of Engineering in providing services to the government, the public, and the scientific and engineering communities. The Council is administered jointly by both Academies and the Institute of Medicine. Dr. Ralph J. Cicerone and Dr. C. D. Mote, Jr., are chair and vice chair, respectively, of the National Research Council.

**www.national-academies.org**

ALAN L. PETERSON, Professor and Chief, Division of Behavioral Medicine, Department of Psychiatry, University of Texas Health Science Center, San Antonio

KAROL E. WATSON, Associate Professor, Division of Cardiology, Department of Medicine, University of California, Los Angeles, School of Medicine

*IOM Staff*

**ABIGAIL MITCHELL,** Study Director
**CAROLYN FULCO,** Scholar
**HEATHER COLVIN,** Program Officer (*until July 2012*)
**EMILY MORDEN,** Research Associate (*until May 2013*)
**JONATHAN SCHMELZER,** Research Assistant
**JOSEPH GOODMAN,** Senior Program Assistant
**DORIS ROMERO,** Financial Associate
**NORMAN GROSSBLATT,** Senior Editor
**FREDERICK ERDTMANN,** Director, Board on the Health of Select Populations

*Consultant*

**MIRIAM DAVIS,** Independent Consultant

# Reviewers

This report has been reviewed in draft form by persons chosen for their diverse perspectives and technical expertise in accordance with procedures approved by the National Research Council's Report Review Committee. The purpose of this independent review is to provide candid and critical comments that will assist the institution in making its published report as sound as possible and to ensure that the report meets institutional standards of objectivity, evidence, and responsiveness to the study charge. The review comments and draft manuscript remain confidential to protect the integrity of the deliberative process. We thank the following for their review of the report:

**John F. Ahearne,** Sigma Xi, The Scientific Research Society
**Stephen V. Cantrill,** Denver Health Medical Center
**Ralph G. Dacey,** Washington University School of Medicine
**Jordan Grafman,** Rehabilitation Institute of Chicago
**John B. Holcomb,** US Army Institute for Surgical Research
**Mark S. Humayun,** University of Southern California School of Medicine
**Thomas E. Kottke,** HealthPartners
**Cato T. Laurencin,** University of Connecticut
**Henry Lew,** University of Hawaii at Manoa
**Roger O. McClellan,** Independent Advisor on Toxicology and Human Health Risk
**Richard Miller,** Vanderbilt Medical Center
**Eric J. Nestler,** Mount Sinai School of Medicine

Andrew C. Peterson, Duke University Medical Center
Rosemary Polomano, University of Pennsylvania School of Nursing
Myrna M. Weissman, Columbia University

Although the reviewers listed above have provided many constructive comments and suggestions, they were not asked to endorse the conclusions or recommendations, nor did they see the final draft of the report before its release. The review of the report was overseen by **Michael I. Posner,** University of Oregon, and **David G. Hoel,** Medical University of South Carolina. Appointed by the National Research Council and the Institute of Medicine, respectively, they were responsible for making certain that an independent examination of the report was carried out in accordance with institutional procedures and that all review comments were carefully considered. Responsibility for the final content of the report rests entirely with the authoring committee and the institution.

# Preface

Since the United States began combat operations in Afghanistan in October 2001 and then in Iraq in March 2003, the numbers of US soldiers killed exceed 6,700 and of US soldiers wounded, 50,500.[1] Although all wars since World War I have involved the use of explosives by the enemy, the wars in Afghanistan and Iraq differ from previous wars in which the United States has been involved because of the enemy's use of improvised explosive devices (IEDs). The use of IEDs has led to an injury landscape different from that in prior US wars. The signature injury of the Afghanistan and Iraq wars is blast injury. Numerous US soldiers have returned home with devastating blast injuries, and they continue to experience many challenges in readjusting to civilian life.

Throughout history, theaters of war have created a stimulus for medical innovation—in technology, emergency care, surgery, and therapeutics—and especially during the past half-century the resulting advances in battlefield medicine have dramatically improved outcomes for wounded warriors (see Figure P-1). However, in the case of blast-related injuries in particular, knowledge of clinical manifestations, pathophysiology, means of prevention, and best therapies has lagged behind the understanding of those related to other combat-related traumas. In the late 18th century, Pierre Jars first proposed that changes in air pressure resulting from explosion, "*la*

---

[1] DOD (Department of Defense). 2013. *US Department of Defense Casualty Status*. http://www.defense.gov/news/casualty.pdf (accessed September 1, 2013).

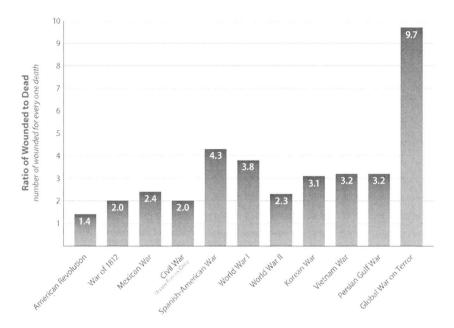

**FIGURE P-1** In contrast with earlier wars, the recent conflicts in Afghanistan and Iraq have witnessed a dramatic increase in the ratio of wounded to deceased soldiers, owing in large part to improvements in battlefield medicine.
SOURCE: Data provided by DOD (Department of Defense). 2013a. *U.S. Military Casualties: GWOT Casualty Summary by Service Component*. https://www.dmdc.osd.mil/dcas/pages/report_sum_comp.xhtml (accessed September 5, 2013); and DOD. 2013b. *Principal Wars in which the United States Participated: U.S. Military Personnel Serving and Casualties*. https://www.dmdc.osd.mil/dcas/pages/report_principal_wars.xhtml (accessed September 5, 2013).

*grande et prompte dilation d'air*," could produce bodily injury or death.[2] That early insight notwithstanding, throughout the 18th and 19th centuries, blast-related injuries were more often attributed, incorrectly, to poisoning from gases released in the explosions rather than to pressure waves.[3]

The modern understanding of blast injury dates from observations on the widespread use of explosives in World War I. Rusca (1915) and Mott (1916) reported that blast explosions could produce fatal injuries without

---

[2]Hill, J. F. 1979. Blast injury with particular reference to recent terrorist bombing incidents. *Annals of the Royal College of Surgeons of England* 61(1):4-11.
[3]Born, C. T. 2005. Blast trauma: The fourth weapon of mass destruction. *Scandinavian Journal of Surgery* 94(4):279-285.

any external signs of trauma,[4,5] Hooker (1924) first described the patho-physiology of blast lung,[6] the high risk of hearing loss due to ear trauma was recognized at about the same time, and *shell shock* became familiar as a term to describe the neurologic and emotional sequelae of blast exposure. The aerial bombing campaigns of World War II and our later entry into the nuclear age stimulated a renewed focus on the many adverse health consequences, acute and chronic, blast injury can have.[7] In recent years, priorities have been shaped by the devastating consequences of IEDs deployed in terrorist attacks against civilians and targeted against military personnel in the current wars in Afghanistan and Iraq.

The committee had two tasks. The first task was to evaluate what is known about health effects of exposure to blast, including the blast waves (the supersonic waves of intense air pressure that follow detonation of an explosive device) and other blast mechanisms, such as blunt-force trauma from projectiles, and to draw conclusions about the strength of the evidence. The committee used an evidence-based approach to identify and evaluate the relevant scientific and medical information on health effects of exposure to blast. Not much information was available in that regard. In particular, research efforts often do not separate blast injuries caused by blast waves from those caused by blunt-force trauma and other mechanisms. Although the committee recognizes that blast injuries are often caused by more than one mechanism and do not occur in isolation and that blast injury typically elicits a secondary multisystem response, it will be important to gain a better understanding of how different blast mechanisms and exposure to repeated blasts directly affect the body. Acute injuries from blast may not be apparent immediately after exposure, especially when people are exposed to the blast waves but not to blunt-force trauma. For example, blast waves alone can affect the nervous system without leaving an obvious acute injury, and blast-related symptoms, such as persistent headache, can develop much later.

The committee's ability to draw conclusions about associations between exposure to blast and health effects, particularly long-term health effects, was severely restricted by the paucity of high-quality information. The second part of its task, therefore, was to develop a research agenda to provide the Department of Veterans Affairs with guidance in addressing the

---

[4]Rusca, F. 1915. Historical article first describing primary blast injury. *Deutcsche Zeitschrift f. Chirurgie* 132:315.

[5]Mott, F. W. 1916. Special discussion on shellshock without visible signs of injury. *Proceedings Royal Society Medicine* 9:i-xxiv.

[6]Hooker, D. R. 1924. Physiological effects of air concussion. *American Journal of Physiology* 67(2):219-274.

[7]Bellamy, R. F., and J. T. Zajtchuk. 1998. *Conventional Warfare. Ballistic, Blast, and Burn Injuries.* Washington, DC: Office of the Surgeon General (Army).

deficiencies in the evidence base. The committee hopes that this research will lead not only to a better understanding of the long-term health effects of exposure to blast but also to improved protective measures for soldiers in the future and to improved treatments for soldiers who experience blast injuries.

The committee is honored to dedicate its report to the men and women who are bravely serving in Middle East battlegrounds, to those who have returned home safely, to our fellow citizens who are recovering from the wounds of war, and to the memory of those who have made the ultimate sacrifice on our behalf. Words cannot convey the depth of our gratitude.

The committee thanks everyone who presented during its public meetings and who provided information that helped us to develop our approach to and thinking about the statement of task. In particular, the committee is grateful to the following: Christopher Crnich, University of Wisconsin School of Medicine and Public Health; Dallas Hack, Combat Casualty Care Research Program, US Army Medical Research and Materiel Command; Mary Lawrence, The Vision Center of Excellence, Department of Defense and Department of Veterans Affairs; Michael Leggieri, Department of Defense Blast Injury Research Program Coordinating Office, US Army Medical Research and Materiel Command; Geoffrey Ling, Defense Advanced Research Projects Agency; Paul Pasquina, Walter Reed National Military Medical Center; Terry Walters, Veterans Health Administration; and Janet Ward, Marina Caroni, and Michael Maffeo, US Army Natick Soldier Research, Development, and Engineering Center.

Finally, the committee thanks the Institute of Medicine staff—Heather Colvin, Carolyn Fulco, Joseph Goodman, Cary Haver, Marc Meisnere, Emily Morden, and Jonathan Schmelzer—who assisted in this effort. In particular, we thank the study director, Abigail Mitchell, who guided the entire process with thoroughness, knowledge, research expertise, and a steady hand at every step along the path.

Stephen L. Hauser, *Chair*
Committee on Gulf War and Health:
Long-Term Effects of Blast Exposures

# Contents

# Abbreviations and Acronyms

| | |
|---|---|
| AbdP | abdominal pressure |
| ANS | autonomous nervous system |
| AOC | alteration of consciousness |
| AOR | adjusted odds ratio |
| AUDIT | Alchohol Use Disorders Identification Test |
| | |
| BAMC | Brooke Army Medical Center |
| BINT | blast-induced neurotrauma |
| BLI | blast lung injury |
| | |
| CAP | compound action potential |
| CDH | chronic daily headache |
| CDP | computerized dynamic posturography |
| CI | confidence interval |
| CNS | central nervous system |
| CPG | clinical practice guideline |
| CTE | chronic traumatic encephalopathy |
| CVP | central venous pressure |
| | |
| DOD | Department of Defense |
| DTI | diffusion tensor imaging |
| | |
| ED | erectile dysfunction |
| EP | endocochlear potential |

| | |
|---|---|
| fMRI | functional magnetic resonance imaging |
| FSH | follicle-stimulating hormone |
| | |
| GCS | Glasgow Coma Scale |
| GHD | growth hormone deficiency |
| GU | genitourinary |
| | |
| HO | heterotopic ossification |
| | |
| ICU | intensive care unit |
| IED | improvised explosive device |
| IOM | Institute of Medicine |
| ISS | injury severity scale |
| | |
| JTTR | Joint Theater Trauma Registry |
| | |
| LH | luteinizing hormone |
| LOC | loss of consciousness |
| LUTS | lower urinary tract symptoms |
| | |
| MDR | multidrug resistance |
| MPO | myeloperoxidase |
| MRI | magnetic resonance imaging |
| mRNA | messenger ribonucleic acid |
| | |
| NACA | N-acetylcysteine amide |
| NAS | National Academy of Sciences |
| NNMC | National Naval Medical Center |
| | |
| OEF | Operation Enduring Freedom |
| OIF | Operation Iraqi Freedom |
| OND | Operation New Dawn |
| OPTIC | Optometry Polytrauma Inpatient Clinic |
| OR | odds ratio |
| | |
| PBI | primary blast injury |
| PFT | pulmonary function test |
| PICS | post-intensive-care syndrome |
| PL | Public Law |
| PNS | VA polytrauma network site |
| PRC | VA polytrauma rehabilitation center |
| PTA | posttraumatic amnesia |

| | |
|---|---|
| PTN | pentaerythritol tetranitrate |
| PTSD | posttraumatic stress disorder |
| | |
| RR | relative risk |
| | |
| SD | standard deviation |
| SimLEARN | VA Simulation Learning, Education and Research Network |
| SM-MHC | smooth muscle myosin heavy chain |
| | |
| TBI | traumatic brain injury |
| ThorP | thoracic pressure |
| TM | tympanic membrane |
| | |
| UK | United Kingdom |
| USAISR | US Army Institute of Surgical Research |
| | |
| VA | Department of Veterans Affairs |
| VHA | Veterans Health Administration |
| VSMC | vascular smooth muscle cell |
| | |
| WRAMC | Walter Reed Army Medical Center |

# Summary

The wars in Iraq and Afghanistan have become known for the enemy's reliance on improvised explosive devices (IEDs). It has been estimated that explosive weaponry accounts for 75% of all US military casualties.[1] Since 2001, about 1,380 US soldiers in the Afghanistan War have been killed in action and 9,813 wounded in action because of IEDs. From March 2003 to November 2011, about 2,209 US soldiers in the Iraq war have been killed in action and 21,743 wounded in action due to IEDs. [2,3] Note that those numbers reflect only service members who have been killed or wounded in action; it is likely that many others are exposed to blast in the combat environment but do not require immediate medical attention and, therefore, are not reflected in the numbers reported.

Explosions may cause five major patterns of injury—primary, secondary, tertiary, quaternary, and quinary. Primary blast injury is caused by the blast wave itself, secondary injury is caused by fragments of debris propelled by the explosion, tertiary injury is due to the acceleration of the body or part of the body by the blast wave or blast wind, quaternary injuries include all other injuries directly caused by a blast but not classified by another mechanism (for example, burns, toxic-substance exposures,

---

[1]Belmont, P. J., A. J. Schoenfeld, and G. Goodman. 2010. Epidemiology of combat wounds in Operation Iraqi Freedom and Operation Enduring Freedom: Orthopaedic burden of disease. *Journal of Surgical Orthopaedic Advances* 19(1):2-7.

[2]iCasualties. 2013. *OEF Fatalities.* http://icasualties.org/oef (accessed September 5, 2013).

[3]Defense Manpower Data Center. 2013. *Global War on Terrorism Casualties by Reason.* http://siadapp.dmdc.osd.mil/personnel/CASUALTY/gwot_reason.pdf (accessed September 1, 2013).

and psychologic trauma), and quinary injuries are illnesses or diseases that result from chemical, biologic, or radiologic substances released by a bomb.

The Department of Veterans Affairs (VA) is concerned about the long-term health effects of exposure to blast. Therefore, it asked that the Institute of Medicine (IOM) conduct a study to assess the relevant scientific information and draw conclusions regarding the strength of the evidence of an association between exposure to blast and health effects. The IOM also was asked to make recommendations for future research on the topic. The IOM appointed the Committee on Gulf War and Health: Long-Term Effects of Blast Exposures to address that task. The specific charge to the committee states that

> the IOM shall comprehensively review, evaluate, and summarize the available scientific and medical literature associated with the multisystem response to blast exposures and subsequent acute and long-term health consequences among Gulf War Veterans. In making determinations, the committee shall consider
>
> a. The strength of scientific evidence, the replicability of results, the statistical significance of results, and the appropriateness of the scientific methods used to detect the association;
> b. In any case where there is evidence of an apparent association, whether there is reasonable confidence that the apparent association is not due to chance, bias, or confounding;
> c. The increased risk of illness among human or animal populations exposed to blast injuries;
> d. Whether a plausible biological mechanism or other evidence of a causal relationship exists between exposure to blast and long-term systemic adverse health effects;
> e. Whether type of blast (for example, shaped blast wave vs diffuse) is associated with injury pattern; and
> f. Whether improvements in collective and personal blast protection are associated with diminished blast injury.
>
> In evaluating the long-term health effects of blast exposures among Gulf War Veterans, the committee should look broadly for relevant information. Information sources to pursue could include but are not limited to
>
> a. Published peer-reviewed literature related to blast injuries among the 1991 Gulf War Veteran population;
> b. Published peer-reviewed literature related to blast injuries in active-duty service members and veterans who served in the Iraq and Afghanistan wars, and other conflicts as appropriate;
> c. Published peer-reviewed literature related to blast injuries among similar populations such as allied military personnel; and
> d. Published peer-reviewed literature related to blast injuries in other populations.

## THE GULF WAR AND HEALTH SERIES

The present volume is part of an IOM series on health effects related to military service during wartime. The series began in 1998 when, in response to the growing concerns of ill Gulf War veterans, Congress passed two laws: Public Law (PL) 105-277, the Persian Gulf War Veterans Act, and PL 105-368, the Veterans Programs Enhancement Act. Those laws directed the secretary of veterans affairs to enter into a contract with the National Academy of Sciences to review and evaluate the scientific and medical literature regarding associations between illness and exposure to toxic agents, environmental or wartime hazards, and preventive medicines or vaccines associated with Gulf War service and to consider the resulting conclusions when making decisions about compensation. The study was assigned to the IOM, and eight volumes have been published.[4]

The legislation did not preclude an IOM recommendation or a VA request for additional studies, particularly as subjects of concern arise. For example, VA's request that the IOM consider whether there is an increased risk of amyotrophic lateral sclerosis in all veteran populations resulted in the report *Amyotrophic Lateral Sclerosis in Veterans*; an examination of all health effects in veterans deployed to the 1991 Persian Gulf War irrespective of specific exposures resulted in *Gulf War and Health, Volume 4: Health Effects of Serving in the Gulf War*; and another VA request regarding the long-term effects of traumatic brain injury resulted in *Gulf War and Health, Volume 7: Long-Term Consequences of Traumatic Brain Injury*. The present volume grew out of discussions with VA over concern about blast injuries and the potential long-term effects of being exposed to a blast.

## HOW THE COMMITTEE APPROACHED ITS CHARGE

The committee was charged with conducting a review of the scientific literature on the association between blast and long-term health effects. The charge did not specify the type of blast injury—primary, secondary, tertiary, quaternary, and quinary—and, therefore, the committee did not attempt to limit its review to any mechanism of blast injury. In fact, many of the studies reviewed by the committee, particularly epidemiologic studies,

---

[4]*Gulf War and Health, Volume 1: Depleted Uranium, Pyridostigmine Bromide, Sarin, Vaccine; Gulf War and Health, Volume 2: Insecticides and Solvents; Gulf War and Health, Volume 3: Fuels, Combustion Products, and Propellants; Gulf War and Health, Volume 4: Health Effects of Serving in the Gulf War; Gulf War and Health, Volume 5: Infectious Diseases; Gulf War and Health, Volume 6: Physiologic, Psychologic, and Psychosocial Effects of Deployment-Related Stress; Gulf War and Health, Volume 7: Long-Term Consequences of Traumatic Brain Injury; and Gulf War and Health, Volume 8: Update of Health Effects of Serving in the Gulf War.*

did not specify the mechanism of exposure (that is, the reported exposure was to blast generally). The review included all relevant studies of blast in any population (military, occupational, and other) and health outcomes. Thus, the committee reviewed all papers that provided information on blast and health outcomes. By examining the full array of evidence of health outcomes in different populations, the committee asked the question, Can sustaining a blast be associated with a specific health outcome?

Several literature searches were performed in 2012 and 2013 in an effort to keep current with the relevant science. The committee reviewed more than 12,800 titles and abstracts of scientific and medical articles related to blast and health outcomes. It also reviewed the full text of about 400 peer-reviewed journal articles, many of which are described in this report.

After obtaining the full-text articles, the committee needed to determine which studies to include in its evaluation. To accomplish that task, the committee developed inclusion guidelines. Studies were categorized as primary or supportive or were excluded from further examination. Primary studies had greater methodologic rigor and so provided the strongest evidence on health outcomes of blast exposure. For many health outcomes, no primary studies were identified; in these cases, supportive studies necessarily guided the committee's determinations. Many of the studies reviewed by the committee had limitations that are commonly encountered in epidemiologic studies, including a lack of representative sample, selection bias, lack of control for potential confounding factors, self-reports of exposure and health outcomes, and outcome misclassification. Because of the inadequacy of epidemiologic literature that can inform understanding of long-term outcomes of exposure to blast, the committee relied heavily on the literature to assess the strength of the evidence on acute effects and on the collective clinical knowledge and expertise of the committee members to draw conclusions regarding the plausibility of the long-term outcomes. Some of the long-term outcomes are obvious and well documented as consequences of the acute injuries; others will require additional research studies to understand the long-term consequences of exposure specifically to blast.

To express its judgment of the available data clearly and precisely, the committee agreed to use the categories of association that have been established and used by previous committees on Gulf War and health and other IOM committees that have evaluated vaccine safety, effects of herbicides used in Vietnam, and indoor pollutants related to asthma. Those categories of association have gained wide acceptance over more than a decade by Congress, government agencies (particularly VA), researchers, and veterans' groups. The five categories in Box S-1 describe different levels of association and sound a recurring theme: the validity of an association is likely to vary to the extent to which common sources of spurious associations can

---

**BOX S-1**
**The Categories of Association**

**Sufficient Evidence of a Causal Relationship**
Evidence is sufficient to conclude that there is a causal relationship between blast exposure and a specific health outcome in humans. The evidence fulfills the criterion of sufficient evidence of an association (below) and satisfies several of the criteria used to assess causality: strength of association, dose–response relationship, consistency of association, temporal relationship, specificity of association, and biologic plausibility.

**Sufficient Evidence of an Association**
Evidence is sufficient to conclude that there is a positive association; that is, a consistent association has been observed between blast exposure and a specific health outcome in human studies in which chance and bias, including confounding, could be ruled out with reasonable confidence as an explanation for the observed association.

**Limited/Suggestive Evidence of an Association**
Evidence is suggestive of an association between blast exposure and a specific health outcome in human studies but is limited because chance, bias, and confounding could not be ruled out with reasonable confidence.

**Inadequate/Insufficient Evidence of an Association**
Evidence is of insufficient quantity, quality, consistency, or statistical power to permit a conclusion regarding the existence of an association between blast exposure and a specific health outcome in humans.

**Limited/Suggestive Evidence of *No* Association**
Evidence from several adequate studies is consistent in not showing a positive association between blast exposure and a specific health outcome. A conclusion of no association is inevitably limited to the conditions and length of observation in the available studies. The possibility of a very small increase in risk of the health outcome after exposure to blast cannot be excluded.

---

be ruled out as the reason for the observed association. Accordingly, the criteria for each category express a degree of confidence that is based on the extent to which sources of error were reduced. The committee discussed the evidence and reached consensus on the categorization of the evidence on each health outcome.

## SUMMARY OF CONCLUSIONS

The committee's conclusions on human health outcomes of exposure to blast and on the effectiveness of blast protection are summarized below. It is important to note that although the information here is presented by individual organ systems and other specific outcomes, exposure to blast often leads to polytrauma (multiple traumatic injuries) and a multisystem response.

### Human Health Outcomes

The committee focused its formal conclusions (below) on long-term adverse health outcomes, particularly those not necessarily caused by a severe or obvious acute injury. Acute injuries to each organ system from exposure to blast are summarized in Chapter 4.

*Sufficient Evidence of a Causal Relationship*

- Penetrating eye injuries resulting from exposure to blast and permanent blindness and visual impairment (visual acuity of 20/40 or worse).
- Some long-term effects on a genitourinary organ—such as hypogonadism, infertility, voiding dysfunction, and erectile dysfunction—associated with severe injury, which is defined as a complete structural and functional loss that cannot be reconstructed.

*Sufficient Evidence of an Association*

- Development of posttraumatic stress disorder (PTSD). The association may be related to direct experience of blast or to indirect exposure, such as witnessing the aftermath of a blast or being part of a community affected by a blast.
- Endocrine dysfunction (hypopituitarism and growth hormone deficiency) in cases of severe or moderate blast-related traumatic brain injury (TBI).
- Postconcussive symptoms and persistent headache in cases of mild blast TBI.
- In non-blast severe or moderate TBI, permanent neurologic disability, including cognitive dysfunction, unprovoked seizures, and headache. These associations also are known outcomes in TBI studies that included blast and non-blast mechanisms considered together. It is plausible that severe or moderate blast TBI is simi-

larly associated with permanent neurologic disability even though studies that specifically addressed blast TBI are lacking.
- Long-term dermal effects, such as cutaneous granulomas.

*Limited/Suggestive Evidence of an Association*

- Chronic traumatic encephalopathy with progressive cognitive and behavioral decline in cases of recurrent blast TBI.
- Long-term effects on the tympanic membrane and auditory thresholds.
- Major limb injuries, including amputations, resulting from exposure to blast and long-term outcomes for the affected limb and for the cardiac system.
- Acute gastrointestinal perforations and hemorrhages, and solid-organ laceration, all of which can have long-term consequences.
- Long-term consequences for the musculoskeletal system, including heterotopic ossification in amputated limbs and osteoarthritis.
- Long-term complications of burns.

*Inadequate/Insufficient Evidence of an Association*

- Tinnitus and long-term effects on central auditory processing.
- Long-term effects on balance dysfunction and vertigo.
- Long-term effects on vision in cases of acute nonpenetrating eye injuries.
- Long-term effects on cardiovascular function, such as accelerated atherosclerosis.
- Long-term effects on pulmonary function, respiratory symptoms, and exercise limitation.
- Long-term effects after acute blast lung injury.
- Long-term gastrointestinal outcomes in the absence of serious acute injury.
- Long-term effects associated with partial injury (defined as incomplete structural and functional loss that can be reconstructed) to a genitourinary organ.
- Long-term effects of infections.

*Additional Conclusions*

On the basis of its evaluation, the committee drew several additional conclusions related to adverse health effects of exposure to blast:

- There is sufficient evidence of a substantial overlap in the symptoms of mild TBI and PTSD exposure to blast, and there is limited/suggestive evidence that most of the shared symptoms are accounted for by PTSD and not a direct result of TBI alone.
- There is inadequate/insufficient evidence to assess the direct contribution of blast to depression, substance-use disorders, and chronic pain; however, the association of PTSD with these disorders is well established.
- There is limited/suggestive evidence that diffuse brain injury with swelling may be more likely after blast than in relation to other mechanisms that lead to TBI.

### Blast Protection

The committee was asked to consider whether improvements in collective and personal blast protection are associated with diminished blast injuries. After evaluating the literature on this topic, the committee concludes

- That there is sufficient evidence of an association between the use of personal protective equipment, including interceptive body armor and eye protection, and prevention of blunt and penetrating injuries caused by exposure to blast.
- That there is inadequate/insufficient evidence to determine whether there is an association between the use of current personal protective equipment and prevention of primary blast-induced (non-impact-induced) injuries.

### RECOMMENDATIONS

As the committee evaluated the available evidence on health effects of exposure to blast, it identified a number of gaps in the evidence base. Filling the data gaps is important for advancing the understanding of how blast affects humans in the short term and the long term. A fundamental feature of exposure to blast is that it can result in complex, multisystem injuries. Attention to those complexities has often been lacking in research studies. *It is important that research on blast emphasize multisystem injury patterns and seek to understand the clinical importance of cross-system interactions.*

Below are the committee's recommendations for research that it believes is most likely to provide VA with knowledge that can be used to inform decisions on how to prevent blast injuries, how to diagnose them effectively, and how to manage, treat, and rehabilitate victims of battlefield traumas in the immediate aftermath of a blast and in the long term.

VA can begin to improve the diagnosis of and treatment for blast injuries, particularly in the case of health outcomes of which there is at least sufficient evidence of an association with exposure to blast (see above). The first step for VA should be to evaluate approaches that are already in place to detect, treat for, and rehabilitate after blast injuries.

**Recommendation 5-1. The Department of Veterans Affairs should conduct a rigorous evaluation to determine whether current approaches for detecting, treating for, and rehabilitating after health outcomes of blast exposure are adequate.**

A limitation of nearly all the studies evaluated by the committee was inadequate information about the exposure to blast. Most of the studies used self-reported exposure data rather than objective measures. Obtaining accurate, objective measurement of exposure to blast is essential for understanding the mechanisms of injury from blast.

**Recommendation 5-2. The Department of Defense should develop and deploy a system that measures essential components of blast and characteristics of the exposure environment, that records and stores the collected information, and that links individual blast-exposure databases with self-reported information and with demographic, medical, and operational data.**

Identifying blast injuries in service members, particularly injuries that are not acutely severe and may go undetected for long periods, poses a major challenge in both clinical and research settings. The ability to define biomarkers of blast injury that could serve as surrogates of exposure would constitute a substantial advance in the study of long-term outcomes of exposure to blast.

**Recommendation 5-3. The Department of Veterans Affairs should conduct epidemiologic and mechanistic studies to identify biomarkers of blast injury.**

The committee identified substantial gaps in much of the published research on blast injuries. The gaps include inadequately powered data sets, incomplete control populations, and poor study designs; an absence of combat-relevant expertise in blast on the research team; and a need to refine and advance preclinical models so that they can predict long-term multisystem effects of blast injuries in humans adequately. Greater collaboration within and among institutions will expand the expertise of research teams and help to fill the gaps, and this approach should be considered a strength, not a limitation, with respect to VA funding priorities.

Recommendation 5-4. To support innovation and improve the state of blast science, the Department of Veterans Affairs should develop opportunities for multidisciplinary research collaborations that cross institutional barriers between the Veterans Health Administration, the Department of Defense, and other institutions.

To assist VA and other researchers in improving the design of future studies, the committee offers several additional recommendations. It also notes that it is important that all studies use a standardized definition of blast exposure once it has been developed.

Recommendation 5-5. The Department of Veterans Affairs should conduct research on acute and long-term consequences of blast injury involving all service members and veterans, not only users of the Veterans Health Administration.

Recommendation 5-6. The Department of Veterans Affairs should create a registry of blast-exposed (not only blast-injured) service members to serve as a foundation for long-term studies.

Recommendation 5-7. The Department of Veterans Affairs should use existing military records to identify a cohort of service members who served in the Iraq and Afghanistan wars to enroll in a prospective study of the long-term effects of blast on health and rehabilitation. The cohort should not be limited to service members who are known to have been exposed to blast.

Recommendation 5-8. The Department of Veterans Affairs should identify and use as a resource existing longitudinal cohort studies on populations that include blast-exposed service members and veterans. This resource may include information from existing ancillary studies of these cohorts to improve the detection and measurement of adverse long-term health outcomes of blast exposure.

Recommendation 5-9. The Department of Veterans Affairs should create a database that links Department of Defense records (particularly records that identify blast-injured service members) to records in the Veterans Health Administration, active-duty military treatment facilities, and TRICARE (the Department of Defense health care program) to facilitate identification of long-term health care needs after blast injury.

Recommendation 5-10. The Department of Veterans Affairs should conduct case-control studies of select adverse outcomes to test for the potential contribution of blast to them.

Knowledge of predictors of increased risk of health conditions associated with blast exposure makes it possible for service members who are at increased risk to be assigned to duties that avoid or minimize particular exposures or to receive prophylactic treatment and rehabilitation. Screening tests conducted on entry into the military (not only before deployment) should be helpful in gathering information on predictors of increased risk of blast injury.

Recommendation 5-11. The Department of Defense should determine whether existing screening tests administered during the physical examination conducted on enlistment can be used to measure susceptibility to blast injury, and if additional screening tests might be helpful in determining whether a service member has an increased susceptibility to blast injury.

As part of its charge, the committee was asked to provide recommendations on disseminating information about the health effects of blast exposure throughout VA for the purpose of improving care and benefits provided to veterans.

Recommendation 5-12. The Department of Veterans Affairs should build on its existing educational and communications infrastructure to educate its clinicians and other health care team members further about the health effects of blast exposure. Specific actions should be taken to

- Develop clinical practice guidelines for blast-related injuries other than traumatic brain injury and posttraumatic stress disorder. The guidelines should be developed in collaboration with the Department of Defense and ideally would be used by both departments.
- Expand the focus of the Polytrauma and Blast-Related Injuries Quality Enhancement Research Initiative to include injuries other than traumatic brain injury and posttraumatic stress disorder. Blast injuries and rehabilitation after them should be viewed through a wide clinical lens.
- Offer continuing education credit courses on blast injury through the Simulation Learning, Education and Research Network and other relevant educational forums.

- Convene periodic state-of-the-science conferences (for example, every 2 or 3 years) on the health effects of blast injuries. Such conferences would be convened ideally in collaboration with the Department of Defense, and possibly with selected professional associations, and the conference proceedings would be published (for example, in special issues or supplements of professional journals).
- Establish a blast-injury literature clearinghouse or information repository that could be used as a resource for clinicians and researchers. It should be a joint effort of the Department of Veterans Affairs and the Department of Defense.
- Use such mechanisms as the Patient Aligned Care Team, clinical champions, and learning networks to educate Department of Veterans Affairs health care teams about the health effects of blast exposure.
- Encourage clinicians to ask veterans specifically about exposure to blasts. Develop standard screening questions specific to veterans' exposures to blast for integration into the Department of Veterans Affairs electronic health record and as part of veterans' military histories. The screening questions should be listed on the military health history pocket card.

# 1

# Introduction

The first Persian Gulf War, known as Operation Desert Storm, was an offensive that followed the August 1990 Iraqi invasion of Kuwait and was led by US and coalition troops in January 1991. The war was over on February 28, 1991, and an official cease-fire was signed in April 1991. The last US troops who participated in the ground war returned home on June 13, 1991. In all, about 697,000 US troops had been deployed to the Persian Gulf during the conflict. That war resulted in few injuries and deaths among coalition forces, but returning veterans soon began to report numerous health problems that they believed were associated with their service in the gulf. Those veterans were not exposed to blast but were potentially exposed to numerous biologic and chemical agents, including vaccinations and other prophylactic medications, nerve agents, depleted uranium, pesticides, solvents, combusted and uncombusted fuels, dust exposure, and burning waste.

On October 7, 2001, the United States began combat operations in Afghanistan in response to the September 11, 2001, terrorist attacks. The war in Afghanistan is also referred to as Operation Enduring Freedom (OEF). On March 20, 2003, the United States became engaged in military operations in Iraq. The Iraq War, also referred to as Operation Iraqi Freedom (OIF), and OEF have been fundamentally different from the first Gulf War in the number of troops deployed, in multiple deployments, in its duration, in the type of warfare, and in the numbers of deaths and injuries, particularly brain injuries. On September 1, 2010, OIF was renamed Operation New Dawn (OND) (Secretary of Defense Memorandum, February 17, 2010). As of September 2013, those wars have resulted in the deployment of about 2.2 million troops; there have been 2,266 US fatalities in OEF and 4,489 in OIF and OND. The numbers of wounded US troops exceed 19,250 in Afghanistan and 32,000 in Iraq (DOD, 2013). In addition to deaths and morbidity, the operations have unforeseen consequences for military personnel that are not yet fully understood.

## STUDY ORIGIN

In 1998, in response to the growing concerns of ill Gulf War veterans, Congress passed two laws: Public Law (PL) 105-277, the Persian Gulf War Veterans Act, and PL 105-368, the Veterans Programs Enhancement Act. Those laws directed the secretary of veterans affairs to enter into a contract with the National Academy of Sciences (NAS) to review and evaluate the scientific and medical literature regarding associations between illness and exposure to toxic agents, environmental or wartime hazards, and preventive medicines or vaccines related to Gulf War service and to consider the NAS conclusions when making decisions about compensation. The study was assigned to the Institute of Medicine (IOM), and several volumes have been published.[1] Several of the volumes address the concerns of not only the 1991 Gulf War veterans but also the veterans of the Iraq and Afghanistan wars.

The legislation did not preclude an IOM recommendation or a Department of Veterans Affairs (VA) request for additional studies, particularly as subjects of concern arise. For example, VA's request that the IOM consider whether there is an increased risk of amyotrophic lateral sclerosis in all veteran populations resulted in the report *Amyotrophic Lateral Sclerosis in Veterans* (IOM, 2006a); an examination of all health effects in veterans deployed to the 1991 Persian Gulf War irrespective of specific exposures resulted in *Gulf War and Health, Volume 4: Health Effects of Serving in the Gulf War* (IOM, 2006b); and a VA request regarding the long-term effects of traumatic brain injury (TBI) resulted in *Gulf War and Health, Volume 7: Long-Term Consequences of Traumatic Brain Injury* (IOM, 2009). The present volume grew out of discussions with VA over concern about blast injuries and the potential long-term effects of being in a blast.

---

[1]*Gulf War and Health, Volume 1: Depleted Uranium, Pyridostigmine Bromide, Sarin, Vaccines* (IOM, 2000); *Gulf War and Health, Volume 2: Insecticides and Solvents* (IOM, 2003); *Gulf War and Health, Volume 3: Fuels, Combustion Products, and Propellants* (IOM, 2005); *Gulf War and Health, Volume 4: Health Effects of Serving in the Gulf War* (IOM, 2006); *Gulf War and Health, Volume 5: Infectious Diseases* (IOM, 2006); *Gulf War and Health, Volume 6: Physiologic, Psychologic, and Psychosocial Effects of Deployment-Related Stress* (IOM, 2008); *Gulf War and Health, Volume 7: Long-Term Consequences of Traumatic Brain Injury* (IOM, 2009); and *Gulf War and Health, Volume 8: Update of Health Effects of Serving in the Gulf War* (IOM, 2010).

## BLAST INJURIES

The wars in Iraq and Afghanistan have become known for the enemy's reliance on improvised explosive devices (IEDs) (Champion et al., 2009; Ritenour et al., 2010). It has been estimated that explosive weaponry accounts for about 75% of all US military casualties (Belmont et al., 2010, 2012). Explosive incidents involving IEDs are a worldwide problem. In 2012, the number of terrorist attacks worldwide involving IEDs, including military combat, was 2,451; 2,634 people were killed and 6,601 wounded (CEDAT, 2013).

It is not possible to know precisely the number of military personnel who served in the Iraq and Afghanistan wars and were exposed to blast. However, data that can serve as a surrogate for blast exposure are available and provide a rough estimate of blast-exposed personnel.

A substantial portion of blast exposure during the Iraq and Afghanistan wars comes from IEDs. Since 2001, about 1,380 OEF service members have been killed in action and 11,312 wounded in action because of IEDs. From March 2003 to November 2011, about 2,207 OIF and OND service members have been killed in action and 21,743 wounded in action because of IEDs (DMDC, 2013; iCasualties, 2013). There were limitations in extrapolating those data to overall blast exposure of military personnel of the Iraq and Afghanistan wars. Those numbers refer only to service members who have been killed or wounded in action. The number of service members exposed to blast in the combat environment is probably much higher.

Another means of estimating the number of blast-exposed military personnel is to use data on numbers of personnel who have received TBIs, particularly mild TBIs. Mild TBIs account for nearly 77% of TBIs (187,539 of the total of 244,217 service members who received TBIs) in personnel serving in the Iraq and Afghanistan wars (IOM, 2013). The major cause of TBI in the Iraq and Afghanistan wars is exposure to blast, often from IEDs. Again, this information provides only a rough estimate of blast exposure, and it is probable that the actual number of service members exposed is much higher.

There are five mechanisms by which injuries can occur after exposure to blast. *Primary injury* is the direct result of spallation, implosion, or inertia; these injuries are caused as a sole consequence of the shock wave–body interaction. Their effects are concentrated on regions where there is an air or fluid interface with tissue (Wolf et al., 2009). For example, a combination of implosion and spallation forces may cause an air embolus to enter a capillary as a blast wave travels through blood and into a capillary where spalling disrupts the endothelium and implosion causes compressed air to expand (Ho, 2002; Wolf et al., 2009). Organ systems that have greater air–tissue interfaces are more susceptible to primary blast injuries. Auditory injury is the most common, occurring at 35 kilopascal (kPa), compared with pulmonary or intestinal injury, which occurs at 75–100 kPa (Wolf et al., 2009). Overpressure may also affect the central nervous, musculo-skeletal, visual, and cardiovascular systems. And a blast wave may cause a systemic shock that subsides in minutes or hours (Wolf et al., 2009). *Secondary injury* is caused by debris that is displaced by a blast wave or blown by the blast wind. A combination of penetrating or blunt injuries may result, including bruises and lacerations. Fragments or shrapnel may create small puncture wounds. Because fragments travel further than a blast wave, secondary injuries are more common than primary injuries (Wolf et al., 2009). *Tertiary injury* results from the physical displacement of a person by a blast wave or blast wind. A person who is pushed or blown may suffer a variety of injuries, such as head trauma or fractures. Injuries associated with falling buildings—such as head trauma, traumatic asphyxiation, and crush injuries—are considered tertiary injuries (Wolf et al., 2009). *Quartenary injuries*, or miscellaneous injuries, include all other injuries directly caused by a blast but not classified by another mechanism. These injuries may be burns, toxic-substance exposures, and psychologic trauma (Wolf et al., 2009). *Quinary injuries* are illnesses or diseases that result from chemical, biologic, or radiologic substances released by a bomb (Cernak and Noble-Haeusslein, 2010; Plurad, 2011). Chapter 3 describes the mechanisms of blast injury in greater detail.

## CHARGE TO THE COMMITTEE

The charge to the present IOM committee was to examine the strength of the evidence of an association between being exposed to blast and potential long-term health effects. The committee also was asked to make recommendations for future research on the topic. Specifically, the statement of work notes that the IOM

> shall comprehensively review, evaluate, and summarize the available scientific and medical literature associated with the multisystem response to blast exposures and subsequent acute and long-term health consequences among Gulf War veterans.

> In making determinations, the committee shall consider

> a. The strength of scientific evidence, the replicability of results, the statistical significance of results, and the appropriateness of the scientific methods used to detect the association;

> b. In any case where there is evidence of an apparent association, whether there is reasonable confidence that the apparent association is not due to chance, bias, or confounding;

c. The increased risk of illness among human or animal populations exposed to blast injuries;
d. Whether a plausible biological mechanism or other evidence of a causal relationship exists between exposure to blast and long-term systemic adverse health effects;
e. Whether type of blast (for example, shaped blast wave vs diffuse) is associated with injury pattern; and
f. Whether improvements in collective and personal blast protection are associated with diminished blast injury.

In evaluating the long-term health effects of blast exposures among Gulf War Veterans, the committee should look broadly for relevant information. Information sources to pursue could include but are not limited to

a. Published peer-reviewed literature related to blast injuries among the 1991 Gulf War Veteran population;
b. Published peer-reviewed literature related to blast injuries among OEF (Operation Enduring Freedom), OIF (Operation Iraqi Freedom), New Dawn active-duty service members and veterans, and other conflicts as appropriate;
c. Published peer-reviewed literature related to blast injuries among similar populations such as allied military personnel; and
d. Published peer-reviewed literature related to blast injuries in other populations.

## HOW THE COMMITTEE APPROACHED ITS CHARGE

The committee was charged with conducting a review of the scientific literature on the association between blast and long-term health effects. The charge did not specify the type of blast injury—primary, secondary, tertiary, quaternary, and quinary—and, therefore, the committee did not attempt to limit its review to any mechanism of blast injury. In fact, many of the studies reviewed by the committee, particularly epidemiologic studies, did not specify the mechanism of exposure (that is, the reported exposure was to blast generally). Chapter 3 includes a detailed description of the types of blast injury. The review included all relevant studies of blast in any population (military, occupational, and other) and health outcomes. The committee reviewed all papers that provided information about blast and health outcomes. By examining the full array of evidence of health outcomes in different populations, the committee answered the question, Can sustaining a blast be associated with a specific health outcome? It should be remembered that an association between a blast and a health outcome does not mean that all cases of the outcome are related to the blast; in fact, such direct correspondence is the exception rather than the rule in studies of health outcomes in large populations (IOM, 1994).

The committee reviewed more than 12,800 titles and abstracts of scientific and medical articles related to blast and health outcomes. It reviewed the full text of about 400 peer-reviewed journal articles, many of which are described in the present report. The staff performed several searches in 2012 and 2013 in an effort to keep current with the literature.

The details of the committee's approach to its charge, the literature-search strategy, the types of studies that were reviewed, the committee's inclusion criteria, and categories of association are described in Chapter 2.

## ORGANIZATION OF THE REPORT

Chapter 2 summarizes the committee's methods for approaching its charge and details of its literature search. A model of possible long-term consequences of exposure to blast is described. Animal models of blast and experimental data are discussed in Chapter 3. Chapter 4 contains the committee's evaluation of the array of human health effects caused by exposure to blast. It also presents the pros and cons of blast protection and the use of body armor. Finally, Chapter 5 presents the committee's recommendations. Biographic information on the committee members is included in an appendix.

## REFERENCES

Belmont, P. J., A. J. Schoenfeld, and G. Goodman. 2010. Epidemiology of combat wounds in Operation Iraqi Freedom and Operation Enduring Freedom: Orthopaedic burden of disease. *Journal of Surgical Orthopaedic Advances* 19(1):2-7.

Belmont, P. J., Jr., B. J. McCriskin, R. N. Sieg, R. Burks, and A. J. Schoenfeld. 2012. Combat wounds in Iraq and Afghanistan from 2005 to 2009. *Journal of Trauma and Acute Care Surgery* 73(1):3-12.

CEDAT (Centre of Excellence Defence Against Terrorism). 2013. *Annual Terrorism Report 2012*. Turkey: NATO.

Cernak, I., and L. J. Noble-Haeusslein. 2010. Traumatic brain injury: An overview of pathobiology with emphasis on military populations. *Journal of Cerebral Blood Flow and Metabolism* 30(2):255-266.

Champion, H. R., J. B. Holcomb, and L. A. Young. 2009. Injuries from explosions: Physics, biophysics, pathology, and required research focus. *Journal of Trauma: Injury, Infection, & Critical Care* 66(5):1468-1477.

DMDC (Defense Manpower Data Center). 2013. *Global War on Terrorism Casualties by Reason*. http://siadapp.dmdc.osd.mil/personnel/CASUALTY/gwot_reason.pdf (accessed September 1, 2013).

DOD (Department of Defense). 2013. *US Department of Defense Casualty Status*. http://www.defense.gov/news/casualty.pdf (accessed June 18, 2013).

Ho, A. M. H. 2002. A simple conceptual model of primary pulmonary blast injury. *Medical Hypotheses* 59(5):611-613.

iCasualties. 2013. *OEF Fatalities*. http://icasualties.org/oef (accessed September 5, 2013).

IOM (Institute of Medicine). 1994. *Veterans and Agent Orange: Health Effects of Herbicides Used in Vietnam*. Washington, DC: National Academy Press.

IOM. 2006a. *Amyotrophic Lateral Sclerosis in Veterans*. Washington, DC: The National Academies Press.

IOM. 2006b. *Gulf War and Health, Volume 4: Health Effects of Serving in the Gulf War*. Washington, DC: The National Academies Press.

IOM. 2009. *Gulf War and Health, Volume 7: Long-Term Consequences of Traumatic Brain Injury*. Washington, DC: The National Academies Press.

IOM. 2013. *Returning Home from Iraq and Afghanistan: Assessment of Readjustment Needs of Veterans, Service Members, and Their Families*. Washington, DC: The National Academies Press.

Plurad, D. S. 2011. Blast injury. *Military Medicine* 176(3):276-282.

Ritenour, A. E., L. H. Blackbourne, J. F. Kelly, D. F. McLaughlin, L. A. Pearse, J. B. Holcomb, and C. E. Wade. 2010. Incidence of primary blast injury in US military overseas contingency operations: A retrospective study. *Annals of Surgery* 251(6):1140-1144.

Wolf, S. J., V. S. Bebarta, C. J. Bonnett, P. T. Pons, and S. V. Cantrill. 2009. Blast injuries. *Lancet* 374(9687):405-415.

# 2

# Methods

This chapter presents the approach that the committee used to identify and evaluate the literature on health effects of blast exposure. It provides information on how the committee conducted its search of the literature, the types of evidence reviewed, the committee's evaluation guidelines, the limitations of the studies reviewed, and the categories of association that the committee used in drawing conclusions about associations between blast exposure and long-term health effects.

## SEARCH STRATEGY AND IDENTIFICATION OF LITERATURE

To identify the relevant published evidence on health effects of blast exposure, the committee began its work by overseeing extensive searches of the medical and scientific literature, such as published peer-reviewed articles and technical reports. Citation databases searched included MEDLINE, Embase, and the National Technical Information Service. Initial searches identified potentially relevant studies of blast-associated injuries other than traumatic brain injury (TBI) through March 2012. Additional searches for material on TBI due to blast exposure were conducted to retrieve studies from 2007 through June 2012 to capture studies that were not included in the previous Institute of Medicine (IOM) report *Gulf War and Health, Volume 7: Long-Term Consequences of Traumatic Brain Injury* (IOM, 2009). A final search was conducted in March 2013 to identify studies published since the previous searches. The various searches retrieved more than 12,800 potentially useful studies. A manual search of titles and abstracts was conducted to exclude nonrelevant studies. The titles and abstracts of the remaining roughly 1,800 studies were then reviewed again. Scientific reviews and other review articles were manually searched for additional relevant studies. Numerous articles in languages other than English were included in the review and translated as needed. The committee also considered other sources of information, such as non-peer-reviewed reports and meeting summaries from the Department of Defense (DOD) and the Department of Veterans Affairs (VA).

The committee focused its attention on clinical and epidemiologic studies of adults who may have long-term health effects (effects present at least 6 months after exposure) that resulted from a blast exposure. However, studies of immediate effects of blast exposures also were considered because acute effects (effects present immediately after the exposure to a blast that might last for hours to weeks) and subacute effects (effects that occur after acute and before long-term, present for weeks to 6 months) potentially could lead to long-term health effects (see Figure 2-1). Reviewing literature on acute and subacute effects of exposures to blast helped the committee to identify data gaps in the evidence base on long-term health effects.

Review of the roughly 1,800 titles and abstracts led to the identification of about 400 studies for further examination at the full-text level. To determine which studies would be included in the evaluation, the committee developed a set of inclusion guidelines (see page 25). All studies were objectively evaluated without preconceptions about health outcomes or about the existence or absence of associations.

## TYPES OF EVIDENCE

The committee relied primarily on clinical and epidemiologic studies to draw its conclusions about the strength of evidence of associations between blast exposures and long-term health effects. However, animal studies played a critical role in clarifying the mechanism of blast injuries and provided biologic understanding of many of the effects seen in humans.

### Epidemiologic Studies

Analytic epidemiologic studies examine associations between two or more variables. *Predictor variable* and *independent variable* are terms for an exposure to an agent of interest in a human population. *Outcome variable* and *dependent variable* are terms for a health event seen in that population. Outcomes can also include a number of nonhealth results, such as use of services, social changes, and employment changes. A principal objective of epidemiology is to understand whether exposure to a specific agent is associated with disease occurrence or other health outcomes. That is most straightforwardly accomplished in experimental studies in which the investigator controls the exposure and the association between exposure and outcome can be measured directly. In the case of blast exposure studies, however, human experiments that directly examine the association between blast exposure and health outcomes are neither ethically nor practically feasible; instead, the association has to be measured in observational studies, and causality has to be inferred. Although they are commonly used synonymously by the general public, the terms *association* and *causation* have distinct meanings (Alpert and Goldberg, 2007).

There are several possible reasons for associations in observational studies: random error (chance); systematic error (bias); confounding; effect–cause relationships; and cause–effect relationships. A spurious association—the finding of an association that does not exist—can be due to random error or chance, systematic error or bias, or a combination of them. *Random error or chance* is a statistical variation in a measurement taken from a sample of a population that can lead to the appearance of an association when none is present or to the failure to find an association when one is present. *Systematic error or bias* is the result of errors in how a study was designed or conducted. Systematic error can cause an observed value to deviate from its true value and can falsely strengthen or weaken an association or generate a spurious association. *Selection bias* occurs when there has been systematic error in recruiting a study population, which is different from the target population of the study, with the result that the findings cannot be generalized to the target population. *Information bias* results from a flaw in how data on exposure or outcome factors are collected.

Other reasons for finding associations that are incorrect are confounding and effect–cause relationships. *Confounding* occurs when a third variable—termed a confounding variable (or confounder)—is associated with both the exposure and the outcome and leads to the mistaken conclusion that the exposure is associated with the outcome. *Effect–cause relationships* occur when the outcome precedes the exposure; for example, a study might suggest that a particular health outcome was associated with blast exposure when the health condition actually preceded the exposure. In a true association, the exposure precedes the outcome and the association is free of random error, bias, and confounding (or the chance of them has been minimized); finding true associations is the goal of epidemiologic studies.

Detection of associations can be affected by the prevalence of health problems in a given population. Attributing an incremental burden of a disease that is common in a population to a specific exposure can be difficult. However, a small increase in the number of cases of a rare disease in a population can produce an effect that is more apparently attributed to an exposure.

In epidemiologic studies, the strength of an association between exposure and outcome is generally estimated by using prevalence ratios, relative risks (RRs), odds ratios (ORs), correlation coefficients, or hazard ratios, depending on the type of epidemiologic study performed. To conclude that an association exists, it is necessary for the exposure to be followed by the outcome more (or less in the case of a protective exposure) frequently than it would be expected to by chance alone. The strength of an association is typically expressed as a ratio of the frequency of an outcome in a group of participants who have a particular exposure to the frequency in a group that does not have the exposure. A ratio greater than 1.0 indicates that the outcome variable has occurred more frequently in the exposed group, and a ratio less than 1.0 indicates that it has occurred less frequently. Ratios are typically reported with confidence intervals to assess random error. If a confidence interval (95% CI) for a ratio measure (such as an RR or an OR) includes 1.0, an association is said to be not statistically significant; if the interval does not include 1.0, the association is said to be statistically significant.

## Animal Studies

Studies of laboratory animals are essential for understanding mechanisms of action and biologic plausibility and for providing information about possible health effects when experimental research in humans is not ethically or practically possible (NRC, 1991). Such studies permit an injury caused by a blast to be introduced under conditions controlled by the researcher. Mechanism-of-action (mechanistic) studies encompass a variety of laboratory approaches with whole animals and in vitro systems that use tissues or cells from humans or animals.

In deciding on associations between blast exposure and human long-term health effects, the committee used evidence only from human studies; in some cases, however, it examined animal studies as a basis of judgments about biologic mechanism or plausibility.

## INFERRING CAUSALITY

Determining whether a given statistical association rises to the level of causation requires inference (Hill, 1965); that is, causality is inferred, rather than measured directly, in observational studies. In 1965, Austin Bradford Hill, a British statistician, suggested nine criteria that could be used to assess whether an association observed in an observational study might be causal:

- *Strength of association*. A strong association is more likely than a modest association to have a causal component.

- *Consistency.* An association that is observed consistently in different studies is more likely to be causal than one that is not.
- *Specificity.* A factor (or predictor variable) influences specifically a particular outcome or population.
- *Temporality.* A factor must precede an outcome that it is supposed to affect.
- *Biologic gradient (also called dose–response relationship).* An outcome increases monotonically with increasing dose of exposure or according to a function predicted by a substantive theory.
- *Plausibility.* An observed association can be plausibly explained by substantive (for example, biologic) explanations.
- *Coherence.* A causal conclusion should not fundamentally contradict present substantive knowledge.
- *Experiment.* Causation is more likely if evidence comes from randomized experiments.
- *Analogy.* An effect has already been shown for analogous exposures and outcomes.

Not all those criteria are applicable in all cases. For example, as noted above, randomized experiments that expose humans to blast would be not conducted. A strong association as measured by a high (or low) risk or ratio, an association that is found in a number of studies, an increased risk of disease with increasing exposure or a decline in risk after cessation of exposure, and a finding of the same outcome after analogous exposures all strengthen the likelihood that an association seen in epidemiologic studies is causal. Exposures are rarely, if ever, controlled in observational studies, and there can be substantial uncertainty in the assessment of a blast exposure. To assess whether explanations other than causality (such as chance, bias, or confounding) are responsible for an observed association, one must bring together evidence from different studies and apply well-established criteria (Evans, 1976; Hill, 1965; Susser, 1973, 1977, 1988, 1991; Wegman et al., 1997).

## INCLUSION GUIDELINES

After obtaining the roughly 400 full-text articles, the committee needed to determine which studies to include in its evaluation. To do that, the committee developed inclusion guidelines. Box 2-1 includes examples of types of evidence used to categorize a study as primary or supportive (secondary or tertiary). Primary studies had greater methodologic rigor and therefore provided the strongest evidence on long-term health outcomes of blast exposure. For many health outcomes no primary studies were identified; in these cases, supportive studies necessarily guided the committee's determi-

---

**BOX 2-1**
**Inclusion Guidelines**

**Primary**
- Cohort study
- Prospective study
- Objective data related to exposure
- Appropriate control or comparison group
- Minimal selection bias
- Long-term followup (more than 6 months)
- Objective outcome of assessment
- Sound analytic methods, sufficiently powered
- Peer-reviewed in some way

**Secondary**
- Case-control study
- Studies dependent on self-report of exposure or outcome
- Peer-reviewed in some way

**Tertiary**
- Case series or reports
- Peer-reviewed in some way

---

nations. If a study did not meet any of the guidelines, it was excluded from further examination.

A study had to have been published in a peer-reviewed journal or other publication—such as a government report, dissertation, or monograph—and had to include sufficient methodologic details to allow the committee to judge whether it met inclusion guidelines. A primary study had to include an unexposed control or comparison group, had to have sufficient statistical power to detect effects, had to use reasonable methods to control for confounders, and had to report followup data for at least 6 months. A study had to include information that the exposure was to blast. Ideally, there was an independent assessment of the exposure rather than self-reported information. Pre-exposure data were almost certainly not available and, realistically, even cohort studies would begin after exposure. Furthermore, exposure to blast is not routinely objectively measured, so researchers had to rely on self-reported exposures. The committee preferred studies that had an independent assessment of an outcome rather than self-reports of an outcome or reports by family members. It was preferable to have the health effect diagnosed or confirmed by a clinical evaluation, imaging, hospital record, or other medical record. For psychiatric outcomes, standardized interviews were preferred, such as the Structured Clinical Interview for the *Diagnostic and Statistical Manual of Mental Disorders, Fourth Edition, Text Revision*, the Diagnostic Interview Schedule, and the Composite International Diagnostic Interview; similarly, for other outcomes, standardized and validated tests were preferred. The committee recognizes that not all health outcomes have objective measures (for example, tinnitus is identified only through self-reported symptoms), that the gold standard for assessment is different for various outcomes, and that for some outcomes there may be more than one gold standard. Finally, the outcome had to be diagnosed after exposure to blast.

## LIMITATIONS OF STUDIES

Many of the studies reviewed by the committee had limitations that are commonly encountered in epidemiologic studies, including lack of representative sample, selection bias, lack of control for potential confounding factors, self-reports of exposure and health outcomes, and outcome misclassification.

Although prospective, randomized, placebo-controlled studies provide the most robust type of evidence, they have not been conducted on the effects of blast in humans for ethical reasons. Few of the studies reviewed by the committee were prospective cohort studies. Rather, most were retrospective clinical record reviews and case studies and series. Many of the studies were limited by small samples and selection biases (for example, the subjects had been admitted to acute-care settings). Low response rates in studies based on survey data also were a limitation.

Studies often lacked unexposed control groups; they lacked comparisons of blast-exposed with non-blast-exposed subjects. And a number of studies compared cases of mild TBI that were associated with exposure to blast with cases of mild TBI that were not so associated, so mild TBI was a given in these study populations.

Lack of long-term followup was a limitation in most of the studies assessed by the committee. Few studies reported outcomes longer than 6 months after exposure to blast. Finally, many of the studies used self-reported outcome measures instead of objective measures.

Those types of limitations made it challenging for the committee to determine associations between exposure to blast and long-term health effects. Because of the inadequacy of epidemiologic literature that can inform long-term outcomes of exposure to blast, the committee relied heavily on the literature to assess the strength of the evidence on acute effects and on its members' collective clinical knowledge and expertise to draw conclusions regarding the plausibility of long-term outcomes. Some of the long-term outcomes are obvious and well documented as a consequence of the acute injuries. Other end points will require additional research studies to understand the long-term consequences of exposure specifically to blast.

## CATEGORIES OF ASSOCIATION

The committee attempted to express its judgment of the available data clearly and precisely. It agreed to use the categories of association that have been established and used by previous committees on Gulf War and health and other IOM committees that have evaluated vaccine safety, effects of herbicides used in Vietnam, and indoor pollutants related to asthma (IOM, 2000, 2003, 2005, 2006, 2007, 2009). The categories of association have gained wide acceptance over more than a decade by Congress, government agencies (particularly VA), researchers, and veterans groups.

The five categories below describe different levels of association and sound a recurring theme: the validity of an association is likely to vary to the extent to which common sources of spurious associations can be ruled out as the reason for the association. Accordingly, the criteria for each category express a degree of confidence that is based on the extent to which sources of error were reduced. The committee discussed the evidence and reached consensus on the categorization of the evidence for each health outcome (see Chapter 4).

### Sufficient Evidence of a Causal Relationship

Evidence is sufficient to conclude that there is a causal relationship between blast exposure and a specific health outcome in humans. The evidence fulfills the criteria of sufficient evidence of an association (below) and satisfies several of the criteria used to assess causality: strength of association, dose–response relationship, consistency of association, temporal relationship, specificity of association, and biologic plausibility.

### Sufficient Evidence of an Association

Evidence is sufficient to conclude that there is a positive association; that is, a consistent association has been observed between blast exposure and a specific health outcome in human studies in which chance and bias, including confounding, could be ruled out with reasonable confidence as an explanation for the observed association.

## Limited/Suggestive Evidence of an Association

Evidence is suggestive of an association between blast exposure and a specific health outcome in human studies but is limited because chance, bias, and confounding could not be ruled out with reasonable confidence.

## Inadequate/Insufficient Evidence of an Association

Evidence is of insufficient quantity, quality, consistency, or statistical power to permit a conclusion regarding the existence of an association between blast exposure and a specific health outcome in humans.

## Limited/Suggestive Evidence of *No* Association

Evidence from several adequate studies is consistent in not showing a positive association between blast exposure and a specific health outcome. A conclusion of no association is inevitably limited to the conditions and length of observation in the available studies. The possibility of a very small increase in risk of the health outcome after exposure to blast cannot be excluded.

## CONCEPTUAL MODEL OF BLAST INJURIES

In approaching the array of possible long-term consequences of blast injury, the committee found it useful to consider a simple conceptual model that follows service members after exposure to a blast. The model (below) demonstrates examples of long-term consequences of blast but does not depict every possible pathway.

Exposure of a service member to a blast can have several outcomes, at least in theory. Some of the outcomes are depicted in Figure 2-1, which shows the extent of disability over time. After exposure to a blast, service members can recover completely with no lasting injuries, clinical or subclinical, as depicted by the green trajectory in Panel A. Such service members do not develop long-term consequences of blast exposure. Service members can sustain acute injuries from blast exposure that results in permanent diseases and disabilities, as shown by the red trajectory in Panel A. Examples are permanent hearing and vision loss and amputation of extremities. The committee reviewed the evidence on those immediate, permanent injuries but, given its charge, focused on long-term consequences of injuries to the body from blast exposures. Service members can sustain injuries from which they seemingly recover but that initiate a constellation of adverse consequences that are not clinically obvious shortly after exposure to blast, being revealed only later, as depicted by the trajectories in Panel C. Subacute effects may

**A**

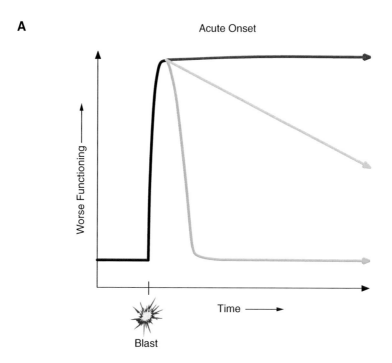

Acute Onset

**B**

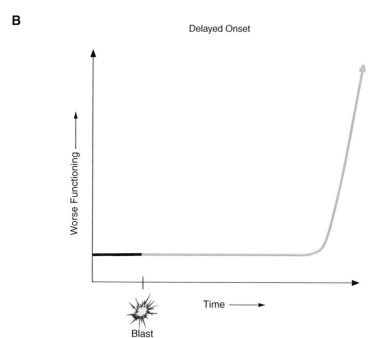

Delayed Onset

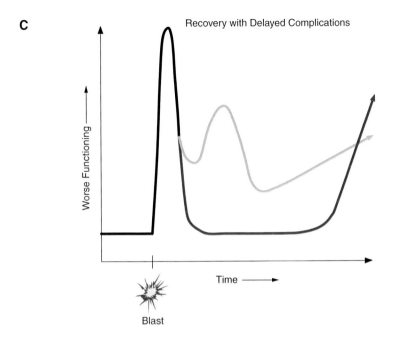

FIGURE 2-1 Examples of possible long-term consequences after exposure to blast. NOTES: Panel A—some service members who are exposed to blast will develop acute injuries and will fully recover within a short period of time, fully recover over a long period of time, or develop chronic diseases and disabilities. Panel B—some service members who are exposed to blast will not experience acute clinically apparent injuries, but may later develop diseases or disabilities, either in the mid- or long term. Panel C—some service members who are exposed to blast will develop acute injuries and then will go on to develop chronic diseases or disabilities even though they had apparently recovered or at least partially recovered in the short term.

be detected in service members shortly after exposure to a blast. Examples of subacute effects might be electroencephalographic changes, headaches, balance impairments, and altered immune responses; these types of effects can be early symptoms of serious long-term consequences, but only sparse data are available.

Service members who do not suffer apparent initial acute injury from blast exposures may be susceptible to long-term consequences (see Panel B). Such service members, in practice in the battlefield, would be indistinguishable from the uninjured. The committee believes that it would be an error, given numerous examples in other fields, to assume that long-term consequences can occur only as a result of clinically detected initial acute injuries caused by blast exposures.

The actual array of possible scenarios is far more complex than that depicted in Figure 2-1. In any service member exposed to blast, multiple organs could be affected and the result can be a constellation of short-term and long-term adverse consequences. The pathways shown in Figure 2-1 probably would intersect, and this would make prediction of long-term consequences challenging. Few data on such interactive effects are available. A key question addressed by the committee later in this report is which long-term consequences can occur only as a result of clinically detectable acute injuries and which can occur even in the absence of clinically detectable acute injuries.

## REFERENCES

Alpert, J. S., and R. J. Goldberg. 2007. Dear patient: Association is not synonymous with causality. *American Journal of Medicine* 120(8):E14-E15.

Evans, A. S. 1976. Causation and disease: The Henle-Koch postulates revisited. *Yale Journal of Biology and Medicine* 49(2):175-195.

Hill, A. B. 1965. Environment and disease: Association or causation. *Proceedings of the Royal Society of Medicine-London* 58(5):295-300.

IOM (Institute of Medicine). 2000. *Gulf War and Health, Volume 1: Depleted Uranium, Pyridostigmine Bromide, Sarin, Vaccines*. Washington, DC: National Academy Press.

IOM. 2003. *Gulf War and Health, Volume 2: Insecticides and Solvents*. Washington, DC: The National Academies Press.

IOM. 2005. *Gulf War and Health, Volume 3: Fuels, Combustion Products, and Propellants*. Washington, DC: The National Academies Press.

IOM. 2006. *Gulf War and Health, Volume 4: Health Effects of Serving in the Gulf War*. Washington, DC: The National Academies Press.

IOM. 2007. *Gulf War and Health, Volume 6: Health Effects of Deployment-Related Stress*. Washington, DC: The National Academies Press.

IOM. 2009. *Gulf War and Health, Volume 7: Long-Term Consequences of Traumatic Brain Injury*. Washington, DC: The National Academies Press.

NRC (National Research Council). 1991. *Animals as Sentinels of Environmental Health Hazards*. Washington, DC: National Academy Press.

Susser, M. 1973. *Causal Thinking in the Health Sciences: Concepts and Strategies of Epidemiology*. New York: Oxford University Press.

Susser, M. 1977. Judgment and causal inference: Criteria in epidemiologic studies. *American Journal of Epidemiology* 105(1):1-15.

Susser, M. 1988. Falsification, verification, and causal inference in epidemiology: Reconsideration in the light of Sir Karl Popper's philosophy. In *Causal Inference*, edited by K. J. Rothman. Chestnut Hill, MA: Epidemiology Resources. Pp. 33-58.

Susser, M. 1991. What is a cause and how do we know one?: A grammar for pragmatic epidemiology. *American Journal of Epidemiology* 133(7):635-648.

Wegman, D. H., N. F. Woods, and J. C. Bailar. 1997. Invited commentary: How would we know a Gulf War syndrome if we saw one? *American Journal of Epidemiology* 146(9):704-711.

# 3

# Pathophysiology of Blast Injury and Overview of Experimental Data

This chapter reviews what is known about the mechanisms of blast injury. It begins with an explanation of blast physics. Next is a discussion of how blast waves interact with the body directly and indirectly and how exposure to blast can affect multiple systems in the body and can cause systemic effects on the autonomic nervous, vascular, and immune systems. That discussion is followed by a description of models used to study blast-injury mechanisms and the challenges involved in using models. The chapter ends with a summary of the results of experimental studies conducted in blast-exposed animal models. The committee used the information presented here to understand the mechanisms of blast injury, to discern clues about possible long-term health effects in humans, and to help to identify data gaps in the evidence base.

## THE PHYSICS OF BLAST

This section is taken from the Institute of Medicine report *Gulf War and Health, Volume 7: Long-Term Consequences of Traumatic Brain Injury* (IOM, 2009). A blast wave generated by an explosion starts with a single pulse of increased air pressure that lasts a few milliseconds. The negative pressure or suction of the blast wave follows the positive wave immediately (Owen-Smith, 1981). The duration of the blast wave—that is, the time that an object in the path of the shock wave is subjected to the pressure effects—depends on the type of explosive and the distance from the point of detonation (Clemedson, 1956). Table 3-1 summarizes the safety zones—that is, the standoff distances—for various types of bomb explosions.

**TABLE 3-1** Safety Recommendations for Standoff Distances from Different Types of Exploding Bombs

| Container or Vehicle Description | Maximum Explosives Capacity | Lethal Air-Blast Range | Maximum Evacuation Distance | Falling-Glass Hazard |
|---|---|---|---|---|
| Pipe 2 × 12 in | 5–6 lb | | 850 ft (259 m) | |
| Pipe 4 × 12 in | 20 lb | | | |
| Pipe 8 × 24 in | 120 lb | | | |
| Bottle 2 L | 10 lb | | | |
| Bottle 2 gal | 30 lb | | | |
| Bottle 5 gal | 70 lb | | | |
| Boxes or shoebox | 30 lb | | | |
| Briefcase or satchel bomb | 50 lb | | 1,850 ft (564 m) | 1,250 ft (381 m) |
| 1-ft³ box | 100 lb | | | |
| Suitcase | 225 lb | | 1,850 ft (564 m) | 1,250 ft (381 m) |
| Compact sedan | 500 lb in trunk | 100 ft (30 m) | 1,500 ft (457 m) | 1,250 ft (381 m) |
| Full-size sedan | 1,000 lb in trunk | 125 ft (38 m) | 1,750 ft (534 m) | 1,750 ft (534 m) |
| Passenger van or cargo van | 4,000 lb | 200 ft (61 m) | 2,750 ft (838 m) | 2,750 ft (838 m) |
| Small box van | 10,000 lb | 300 ft (91 m) | 3,750 ft (1,143 m) | 3,750 ft (1,143 m) |
| Box van or water or fuel truck | 30,000 lb | 450 ft (137 m) | 6,500 ft (1,982 m) | 6,500 ft (1,982 m) |
| Semitrailer | 60,000 lb | 600 ft (183 m) | 7,000 ft (2,134 m) | 7,000 ft (2,134 m) |

NOTE: Table compiled from several publications of the Advanced Technical Group for Blast Mitigation and Technical Support Working Group.
SOURCE: Reprinted with permission from Charles Stewart, MD, EMDM, MPH (Stewart, 2014).

   The blast wave progresses from the source of the explosion as a sphere of compressed and rapidly expanding gases, which displaces an equal volume of air at a high velocity (Rossle, 1950). The velocity of the blast wave in air may be extremely high, depending on the type and amount of the explosive used. The blast wave is the main determinant of the primary blast injury and consists of the front of high pressure that compresses the surrounding air and falls rapidly to negative pressure. It travels faster than sound and in few milliseconds damages the surrounding structures. The blast wind following the wave is generated by the mass displacement of air by expanding gases; it may accelerate to hurricane proportions and is responsible for disintegration, evisceration, and traumatic amputation of body parts. Thus, a person exposed to an explosion will be subjected not only to a blast wave but to the high-velocity wind traveling directly behind the shock front of the blast wave (Rossle, 1950). A hurricane-force wind traveling about 200 km/h exerts overpressure of only 1.72 kilopascal (kPa) (0.25 psi), but a blast-induced overpressure of 690 kPa (100 psi) that causes substantial lung damage and might be lethal travels at about 2,414 km/h (Owen-Smith, 1981).

   The magnitude of damage due to the blast wave depends on the peak of the initial positive-pressure wave (an overpressure of 414–552 kPa or 60–80 psi is considered potentially lethal), the duration of the overpressure, the medium of the explosion, the distance from the incident blast wave, and the degree of focusing due to a confined area or walls. For example, explosions near or within hard solid surfaces become amplified 2–9 times because of shock-wave reflection (Rice and Heck, 2000). Moreover, victims positioned between the blast and a building often suffer 2–3 times the degree of injury of a person in an open space. Indeed, people exposed to explosion rarely experience the idealized pressure-wave form, known as the Friedlander wave. Even in open-field conditions, the blast wave reflects from the ground, generating reflective waves that interact with the primary wave and thus changing its characteristics. In a closed environment (such as a building, an urban setting, or a vehicle), the blast wave interacts with surrounding structures and creates multiple wave reflections, which, interacting with the primary wave and between each other, generate a complex wave (Ben-Dor et al., 2001; Mainiero and Sapko, 1996) (see Figure 3-1). Table 3-2 summarizes the effects of different levels of overpressure on material surrounding the explosion and unprotected persons exposed to blast.

   Previous attempts to define the mechanisms of blast injury suggested the involvement of spalling, implosion, and inertial effects as major physical components of the blast-body interaction and later tissue damage (Benzinger, 1950). Spallation is the disruption that occurs at the boundary between two media of different densities; it occurs when a compression wave in the denser medium is reflected at the interface. Implosion occurs

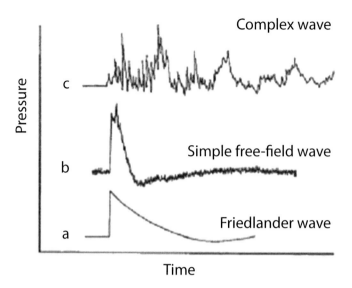

FIGURE 3-1 Explosion-induced shock waves: (a) idealized representation of pressure-time history of an explosion in air; (b) shock wave in open air; (c) complex shock-wave features in closed or urban environment.
SOURCE: Mayorga, 1997. Reprinted with permission from Elsevier Science, Ltd. 2008.

when the shock wave compresses a gas bubble in a liquid medium, raising the pressure in the bubble much higher than the shock pressure; as the pressure wave passes, the bubbles can re-expand explosively and damage surrounding tissue (Benzinger, 1950; Chiffelle, 1966; Phillips, 1986). Inertial effects occur at the interface of the different densities: the lighter object will be accelerated more than the heavier one, so there will be a large stress at the boundary. Recent results suggest that there is a frequency dependence of the blast effects: high-frequency (0.5–1.5 kHz) low-amplitude stress waves target mostly organs that contain abrupt density changes from one medium to another (for example, the air–blood interface in the lungs or the blood–parenchyma interface in the brain), and low-frequency (<0.5 kHz) high-amplitude shear waves disrupt tissue by generating local motions that overcome natural tissue elasticity (for example, at the contact of gray and white brain matter).

**TABLE 3-2** Overpressure Effects on Surrounding Materials and Unprotected Persons

| Pressure, kPa (psi) | Effects on Material | Pressure, kPa (psi) | Effects on Unprotected Person |
|---|---|---|---|
| 0.69–34.47 (0.1–5) | Shatter single-strength glass | 34.47 (5) | Slight chance of eardrum rupture |
| 6.89–13.79 (1–2) | Crack plaster walls, shatter asbestos sheet, buckle steel sheet, failure of wood wall | 103.42 (15) | 50% chance of eardrum rupture |
| 13.79–20.68 (2–3) | Crack cinder-block wall, crack concrete block wall | 206.84–275.79 (30–40) | Slight chance of lung damage |
| 13.79–55.16 (2–8) | Crack brick wall | 551.58 (80) | 50% chance of severe lung damage |
| 34.47–68.95 (5–10) | Shatter car safety glass | 689.48 (100) | Slight chance of death |
| | | 896.32–1,241.06 (130–180) | 50% chance of death |
| | | 1,378.95–1,723.69 (200–250) | Death usual |

SOURCE: Reproduced from *Journal of the Royal Army Medical Corps*, Hunterian lecture 1980: A computerized data retrieval system for the wounds for war: The Northern Ireland casualties. Owen-Smith, M. S., 127(1):31–54, Copyright 1981, with permission from BMJ Publishing Group Ltd.

## ACUTE BLAST–BODY AND BLAST–BRAIN INTERACTIONS

Explosive blast may have five distinct acute effects on the body (see Figure 3-2): The primary blast mechanism causes injuries as sole consequences of the shock wave–body interaction; the secondary blast mechanism is due to the propulsion of fragments of debris by the explosion and their connection with the body, which causes penetrating or blunt injuries; the tertiary blast mechanism is due to the acceleration and deceleration of the body or a part of the body when the energy released by the explosion propels the body or body part (acceleration phase) and then the body or body part stops suddenly on hitting the ground or a surrounding object; the quaternary blast mechanism (not depicted in Figure 3-2) includes flash burns caused by the transient but intense heat of the explosion (Mellor, 1988); and the quinary blast mechanism (not depicted in Figure 3-2) is caused by post-detonation environmental contaminants, such as tissue reactions to fuel,

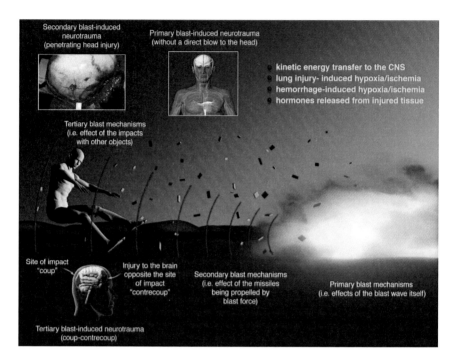

FIGURE 3-2 Complex injurious environment due to blast.
NOTES: Primary blast effects are caused by the blast wave itself (excludes penetrating and blunt-force injury); secondary blast effects are caused by particles propelled by the blast (penetrating or blunt-force injury); tertiary blast effects caused by acceleration and deceleration of the body and its impact with other objects (penetrating or blunt-force [including "coup-contrecoup"] injury). Quaternary and quinary blast effects are not depicted in this figure but are described in the text.
SOURCE: Reprinted with permission from Macmillan Publishers Ltd: *Journal of Cerebral Blood Flow and Metabolism*, Cernak and Noble-Haeusslein, copyright 2010.

metals, and dusts or to bacteria and radiation in dirty bombs (Kluger et al., 2007). Often, especially in the case of moderate to severe blast injuries, the multiple blast effects interact with the body simultaneously; such an injurious environment and related injuries are sometimes called blast-plus (Moss et al., 2009).

When an explosive shock wave strikes a living body, a fraction of the shock wave is reflected and another fraction is absorbed and propagates through the body as a tissue-transmitted shock wave (Clemedson and Criborn, 1955). Different organ and body structures differ in their reactions, but two main general types of tissue response are observed: One is caused by the impulse of the shock wave and is of longer duration, and the other is caused by the pressure variations of the shock wave and is in the form of oscillations or pressure deflections of shorter duration (Clemedson and Pettersson, 1956). For example, Clemedson and colleagues demonstrated that in rabbits exposed to blast, abdominal organs and costal interspaces (that is, spaces between ribs) responded to the impulse of the shock wave, whereas the rib's and the hind leg's response was induced by the pressure variations of the shock wave (Clemedson et al., 1969).

During the interaction between the blast shock wave (the primary blast) and a medium—which could be solid, liquid, gas, or plasma—the energy of the shock wave is absorbed or transformed into the kinetic energy of the medium (Tümer et al., 2013). The kinetic energy, in turn, moves and accelerates the elements of the medium from their resting state with a rate that depends on the density of the medium; this leads to rapid physical movement, displacement, deformation, or rupture of the medium (Chu et al., 2005). Consequently, the main mechanisms of the blast–body interaction and later tissue damage include spallation, implosion, and inertial effects (Richmond et al., 1967). Spallation is a phenomenon that occurs at the boundary between two media of different densities where a compression wave in the denser medium is reflected at the interface. Implosion occurs in a liquid medium that contains a dissolved gas. As the shock wave passes through such a medium, it compresses the gas bubbles, and this leaves the pressure in the bubbles much higher than the shock pressure; after the passage of the pressure wave, the bubbles can re-expand explosively and damage surrounding tissue (Cooper et al., 1991; Richmond et al., 1967, 1968). Inertial effects also occur at the interface of media of different densities: the lighter object will be accelerated more than the heavier one, so there will be a large stress at the boundary (Lu and Wilson, 2003).

In addition to the consequences of the kinetic-energy transfer, recent results suggest that the primary blast effects depend on frequency: High-frequency (0.5–1.5 kHz), low-amplitude stress waves target mostly organs that contain media with contrasting densities (for example, the air–blood interface in the lungs or the blood–parenchyma interface in the brain), and low-frequency (<0.5 kHz), high-amplitude shear waves disrupt tissue by generating local motions that overcome natural tissue elasticity (Cooper et al., 1991; Gorbunov et al., 2004) (for example, at the interface between gray and white brain matter).

## MODIFYING POTENTIAL OF SYSTEMIC CHANGES CAUSED BY BLAST

Because of the complexity of the injurious environment—that is, multiple blast effects that may interact with the body—blast injuries often

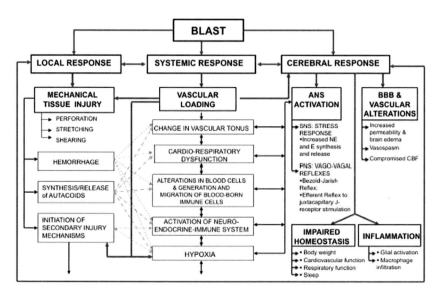

FIGURE 3-3 Simultaneous activation of systemic, local, and cerebral responses to blast exposure and interactive mechanisms that cause or contribute to the blast-induced neurotrauma.
NOTES: ANS = autonomous nervous system; BBB = blood brain barrier; CBF = cerebral blood flow; E = epinephrine; NE = norepinephrine; PNS = parasympathetic nervous system; SNS = sympathetic nervous system.
SOURCE: Cernak, 2010.

involve interwoven mechanisms of systemic, local, and cerebral responses to blast exposure (Cernak et al., 1991, 1996b) (see Figure 3-3). Even when multiorgan responses are mild, systemic changes substantially modify the original organ damage and influence its severity and outcome. Air emboli, activation of the autonomic nervous system (ANS), vascular mechanisms, and systemic inflammation are among the most important systemic alterations that could modify initial injuries due to blast.

### Air Emboli

Air emboli develop as a consequence of the shock wave's passing through media in the body that have different densities: gas, such as air; fluid, such as blood; and solid, such as parenchyma. Experimental studies published by Mason et al. (1971) and Nevison et al. (1971) used an ultrasonic Doppler blood-flow detector in dogs subjected to blast in a shock tube and showed air emboli passing through the carotid artery. The embolus detector showed cyclic release of air emboli: Release occurred over the first 10 seconds after the blast, ceased for a time, and was then noted about 2 minutes and 12 minutes after the blast.

It is noteworthy that the air-emboli release occurred in parallel with a drastic decrease in blood-flow velocity and with seizure that was probably due to hypoxia or anoxia. Similar experimental findings have been described by others (Chu et al., 2005; Clemedson and Hultman, 1954; Kirkman and Watts, 2011) and have been noted in clinical studies (Freund et al., 1980; Tsokos et al., 2003a,b). Indeed, a massive compressed-air embolism of the aorta and multiple air spaces in the interstitium compressing the collecting tubules in the kidneys (Freund et al., 1980) and venous air embolism in the lungs (Tsokos et al., 2003a) were reported in victims of severe blast injuries. It is expected that the rate of the air-emboli release is dependent on the intensity of blast, and the subsequent changes in blood flow and oxygenation concentration are also graded (that is, when the rate of the air-emboli release increases with the increase of blast intensity, the intensity of the pathological changes in blood flow and oxygenation concentration also increases).

### Activation of the Autonomic Nervous System

When the incident overpressure wave (the initial shock wave that brings a sudden increase in atmospheric pressure) is transmitted through the body, it increases the pressure in organs (Clemedson and Pettersson, 1956). The later sudden hyperinflation of the lungs (Cernak et al., 1996b; Zuckerman, 1940) stimulates the juxtacapillary (J) receptors that are located in the alveolar interstitium and innervated by vagal fibers (Paintal, 1969). The resulting vagovagal reflex leads to apnea followed by rapid breathing, bradycardia, and hypotension, which are frequently observed immediately after blast exposure. Moreover, hypoxia and ischemia due to damaged alveoli, air emboli, or a triggered pulmonary vagal reflex can activate a cardiovascular decompressor Bezold-Jarish-reflex, which involves a marked increase in vagal (parasympathetic) efferent discharge to the heart (Zucker, 1986). That effect causes a slowing of the heart (bradycardia), dilation of the peripheral blood vessels, and an ensuing drop in blood pressure, which could contribute further to cerebral hypoxia (Cernak et al., 1996a,b). Axelsson and colleagues (2000) showed in pigs that the blast-induced brief apnea correlated with flattening of the electric activity of the brain. Other experimental studies demonstrated the importance of vagally mediated cerebral effects of blast (Cernak et al., 1996b; Irwin et al., 1999; Ohnishi et al., 2001).

The environment in which an explosion occurs is dramatic and may initiate endocrine mechanisms of the classic flight-and-fight stress response

(Selye, 1976). For example, recent study (Tümer et al., 2013) showed increased expression of the catecholamine-biosynthesizing enzymes tyrosine hydroxylase and dopamine hydroxylase in the rat adrenal medulla and increased plasma concentrations of norepinephrine 6 hours after blast injury. Accumulating experimental and clinical evidence suggests that blast induces alterations in ANS activity: instantaneous triggering of the parasympathetic reflexes followed by neuroendocrine changes due to the activation of the sympathetic nervous system.

### Vascular Mechanisms

One of the most important media for a shock wave's energy transfer is blood. Veins contain about 70% of total human blood volume (including the splanchnic system, which accounts for about 20% of that total), compared with 18% in arteries and only 3% in terminal arteries and arterioles (Gelman, 2008). In general, veins are 30 times more compliant than arteries; splanchnic and cutaneous veins are the most compliant veins and constitute the largest blood reservoirs in the body. Figure 3-4 is a schematic

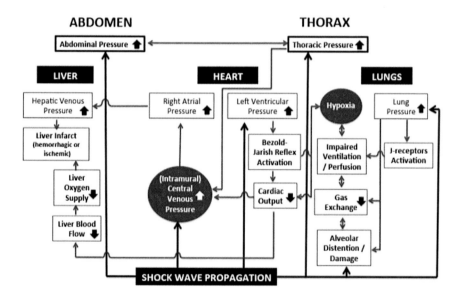

FIGURE 3-4 Overview of vascular mechanisms that are activated by shock-wave propagation through the body, lead to alterations in functions of multiple organs and organ systems, and substantially influence the brain's response to blast.
SOURCE: Created by Ibolja Cernak for the Committee on Gulf War and Health: Long-Term Effects of Blast Exposures.

representation of the consequences of blast-induced pressure changes and their extremely complex interactions, which form several interconnected loops. The transfer of the shock wave's energy to the body not only leads to a sudden increase in both abdominal pressure (AbdP) and thoracic pressure (ThorP) but causes an increase in intramural central venous pressure (CVP). Hypoxia caused by alveolar damage and later by reduced surface for gas exchange, impaired ventilation and perfusion caused by J-receptor activation, or decreased cardiac output due to activation of the Bezold-Jarish reflex all increase pulmonary arterial resistance, which might increase ThorP (Gelman, 2008). An increase in ThorP amplifies the increase in CVP.

Venoconstriction and the mobilization of blood volume depend mainly on the splanchnic circulation, which has a high population of α1- and α2-adrenergic receptors and hence a high sensitivity to adrenergic stimulation (Pang, 2001; Rutlen et al., 1979). Thus, it is likely that the initial sudden drop in systemic arterial pressure caused by blast-induced vagovagal reflexes and the accompanying reduction in the inhibitory influences of the baroreceptors of the carotid sinus and aortic area on the vasomotor center initiate a compensatory increase in sympathetic outflow. The increased sympathetic stimuli constrict venous smooth muscle and lead to mobilization of blood from the splanchnic vasculature toward the heart (Rutlen et al., 1979).

Spasm of the cerebral vasculature has frequently been found in moderate or severe blast-induced traumatic brain injury (TBI)—more often than in patients who have TBI of other origins (for example, impact, fall, or acceleration) (Armonda et al., 2006; Ling et al., 2009). It can develop early, often within 48 hours of injury, and can also be manifested later, typically 10–14 days after exposure. It is noteworthy that although cerebral vasospasm is usually prompted by subarachnoid hemorrhage, that is not required for vasospasm in blast-induced TBI (Magnuson et al., 2012). A recent experimental study of theoretical and in vitro models demonstrated that a single rapid mechanical insult is capable of inducing vascular hypercontractility and remodeling, which are indicative of vasospasm initiation (Alford et al., 2011). Alford and colleagues used in vitro engineered arterial lamellae exposed to high-velocity acute uniaxial stretch to reproduce blast-induced stretch of arterial blood vessels and test whether blast forces can lead to phenotypic switch in vascular smooth muscle cells (VSMCs). The authors measured protein and mRNA expression of two primary markers of contractile VSMCs, smooth muscle myosin heavy chain (SM-MHC) and smoothelin, 24 hours after the injury induction. The results showed that severe (10%) strain decreased expression of smoothelin and decreased mRNA expression of both smoothelin and SM-MHC, suggesting that acute mechanical injury can potentiate a switch away from the contractile phenotype in VSMCs. The findings support a hypothetical scenario in which the shock wave passing through the vasculature interacts with cellular elements of vascular wall (endothelium and vascular smooth muscle) and stimulates synthesis and release of different mediators and modulators. The released biologically active molecules, in turn, cause hypercontractility and later a phenotype switching that potentiates vascular remodeling and cerebral vasospasm (Alford et al., 2011).

### Systemic Inflammation

Blast exposure can activate multiple inflammatory mechanisms (Cernak, 2010). Tissue disruption stimulates synthesis and release of autacoids, biologic factors that act briefly like local hormones near the site of their synthesis. Increased concentrations of prostaglandins, leukotrienes, and cytokines have been found in the blood of blast casualties (Cernak et al., 1999a,b; Surbatovic et al., 2007). The autacoids directly affect a number of stages of immunity and act as feedback modifiers in connecting the early and late phases of the immune response (Melmon et al., 1981). They can stimulate selected migration of cells to an injury site and directly or indirectly modify the turnover of T and B lymphocytes, the production or release of lymphokines, and the activity of T-helper or T-suppressor cells (Khan and Melmon, 1985; Melmon et al., 1981). It has been suggested that inflammatory cells of systemic origin induced by shock-wave propagation through the body contribute substantially to blast-induced inflammation in the brain and related neurodegeneration (Cernak, 2010); the suggestion was supported by experimental data from preclinical models (Valiyaveettil et al., 2013).

Blast exposures have been reported to cause alterations in the neuroendocrine system that involve multiple hypothalamopituitary end axes (Cernak et al., 1999c; Wilkinson et al., 2012). The importance of the immune-neuroendocrine network in injury response and inflammation control is well established (Besedovsky and DelRey, 1996; Chrousos, 1995). It is likely that blast exposure, through multiple interwoven mechanisms, causes a massive perturbation of the central nervous system (CNS) with broad consequences for all aspects of vital functions.

## REQUIREMENTS FOR MODELS OF BLAST-INDUCED INJURY

Regardless of the research questions to be addressed, clinically and militarily relevant blast-injury models should satisfy the following criteria (Cernak and Noble-Haeusslein, 2010):

- the injurious component of the blast is clearly identified and reproduced in a controlled and quantifiable manner.

- the inflicted injury is reproducible and quantifiable and mimics components of human blast injuries.
- the injury outcome—on the basis of morphologic, physiologic, biochemical, and behavioral measures—is related to the chosen injurious component of the blast.
- the mechanical properties—intensity, complexity of blast signature, and duration—of the injurious factor predicts outcome severity.

Compared with the injuries caused by an impact or acceleration–deceleration force, the mechanistic factors underlying blast injuries are extremely complex. Hence, an appropriate and clinically relevant blast-injury model should be based on sufficient knowledge of shock-wave physics and on the characteristics of the injurious environment generated by an explosion and clinical manifestations of resulting injuries. Substantial inter-species differences in responses to blast exposure across different mammalian species make it imperative that research studies of blast effects and the mechanism by which they are produced consider the possible advantages of using species similar in size to humans, and caution should be exercised in extrapolating to humans observations made in rodents and isolated cells and tissues.

## Choice of Models

The design and choice of a specific model depend on the goal of research and the component of clinical CNS injury that one wishes to simulate (Cernak, 2005; Risling and Davidsson, 2012). Given the complex nature of blast injuries, it is obvious that the conditions used in a model to reproduce some aspects of blast injuries should be defined with rigor; otherwise, the results obtained will lack military and clinical relevance and can be dangerously misleading. Indeed, despite the growing literature on experimental blast injuries, the results of studies are difficult to compare because of vast differences in methods and experimental conditions (Panzer et al., 2012). Figure 3-5 is a schematic depiction of the decision-making steps in the process of choosing a model for blast research. First, the researcher should clarify the blast effects to be reproduced. If the choice is primary blast, the researcher should ensure that the animals are fixed so that there will be no blast-induced acceleration of the body and head during the exposure.

In a situation in which the body or head is allowed to move, the injury mechanisms involve both primary and tertiary blast effects, which could introduce difficulties in the proper interpretation of results. Next, a decision should be made about the biologic complexity of the research study because this will dictate the choice of research environment, the means of

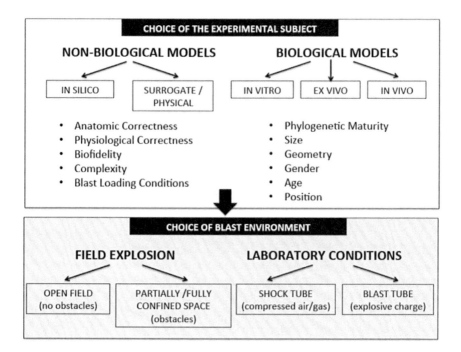

FIGURE 3-5 Factors that influence the choice of blast-injury and blast-induced-neurotrauma models.
SOURCE: Created by Ibolja Cernak for the Committee on Gulf War and Health: Long-Term Effects of Blast Exposures.

generating a shock wave, the choices of models and their positioning, and the length of the experiment. Thus, on the basis of the research question and the complexity, a choice is made between nonbiologic models and biologic models. The nonbiologic models provide an experimental platform for analyzing interactions between blast loading and different types of materials; the information gained is extrapolated to biologic materials at different levels of scaling. The nonbiologic models can be computer simulations and surrogate physical models. Biofidelic models (mechanical models with computerized sensors that mimic particular human characteristics) are helpful for characterizing the physics of the blast-induced mechanical changes in the brain or head. They are made from synthetic materials, such as glass and epoxy or polyurethane. Multiple displacement and pressure sensors molded into the organs' material are used to record biomechanical measures, such as linear and angular acceleration, velocity, displacement, force, torque, and pressure (Desmoulin and Dionne, 2009; Ganpule et al., 2012; Roberts et al., 2012).

Nonbiologic models can be useful in recording biomechanical alterations induced by blast load and suggesting potential consequences, but they are incapable of providing insight into the mechanisms of later physiologic alterations; hence the need for biologic models. The latter models use biologic systems of differing complexity and include in vitro, ex vivo, and in vivo models. In vitro models based on cell cultures can be useful for characterizing cell responses to blast loading in a highly controlled experimental environment (Effgen et al., 2012; Panzer et al., 2012). Ex vivo models use an organ or a segment of a specific tissue, such as brain or spinal cord, taken from the organism and placed in an artificial environment that is more controlled than is possible with in vivo experiments. As with all blast-injury models, applying operationally relevant loading histories is critical for the in vitro and ex vivo models. Only if blast-loading conditions that are realistic and that mimic what would happen at the cellular or tissue level in a person exposed to a militarily relevant blast environment are used can the mechanisms of the energy transfer to the tissue and the resulting biologic response be reliably analyzed (Effgen et al., 2012).

The success of a research study that uses biologic models, especially at the whole-animal level, depends on rigorous selection of the species to be used as experimental models. The choice of animal species depends on the focus of the study (Cernak, 2005). Many investigators have accepted rodent models as the most suitable choice for trauma research. The relatively small size and low cost of rodents permit repetitive measurements of morphologic, biochemical, cellular, and behavioral characteristics that require relatively large numbers of animals; for ethical, technical, and financial reasons, such measurements are less achievable in phylogenetically higher species (Cernak, 2005). However, because of substantially anatomic and physiologic differences, especially in the circulatory and nervous systems, it has been suggested that rodents should not be the sole choice in blast-injury research.

Extensive studies conducted in Albuquerque, New Mexico, and confirmed by British, German, and Swedish findings demonstrated substantial differences in blast tolerance among 15 mammals (Bowen et al., 1968a; Richmond et al., 1967, 1968). Body size–dependent differences in blast tolerance have been explained on the basis of lung density: the lung density in larger species—including humans, monkeys, cats, and dogs—is only about one-half that in smaller species, such as rodents (see Figure 3-6). In contrast, the lung volumes relative to body mass are three times greater in large species than in smaller animals (White et al., 1965). The body size of the animal model is an important consideration for extrapolating to humans; however, size is only one factor to be considered when validating

48

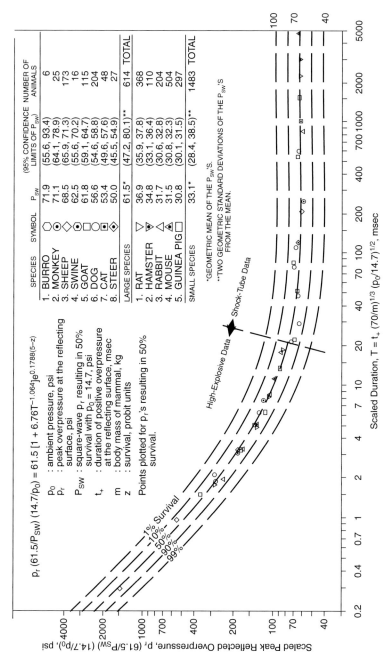

**FIGURE 3-6** Survival curves (24-hour) applicable to sharp-rising blast waves, derived from the analysis of data of 12 mammalian species (excluding guinea pig).
SOURCE: Bowen et al., 1968b.

a model. In addition, substantial interspecies differences in body geometry influence blast–body and blast–head interactions (Bass et al., 2012). The body position of the animal also has an important effect on blast-injury severity. Animals facing an incoming shock-wave front with their chest and abdomen (that is, in the supine position with the shock wave coming from above) provide the most efficient conditions for the shock wave's energy transfer and thus sustain the highest mortality and the most severe injuries (Cernak et al., 2011). In blast-injury modeling, especially when acceleration is included as one of the mechanistic factors, the basic principles of scaling laws should be carefully considered (Bass et al., 2008, 2012). For example, a given blast–head scenario, calculation of the net loading scales for a cross-sectional area of the skull, even if other measures are identical, shows that a specimen 20 times as large would experience one-twentieth the acceleration. However, there are other important anatomic differences between human and animal heads, such as bone volume fraction, trabecular separation, trabecular number, and connectivity density (Bauman et al., 2009; Holzer et al., 2012). Interspecies differences in the structure and arrangement of blood vessels (Vriese, 1904) should also be taken into account in choosing models to reproduce blast injury. For example, the internal carotid artery in lower vertebrates directs the blood to the brain parenchyma through the posterior branch without a contribution from the basilar artery, whereas the two posterior branches in higher vertebrates stem from a single, central branch at the basilar artery (Casals et al., 2011). This anatomical difference could significantly influence the shock-wave propagation through the cerebral vasculature.

It has been shown that phylogenetic maturity has a decisive role in the brain's response to a high-pressure environment (Brauer et al., 1979), and this should be taken into account in planning blast-induced neurotrauma (BINT) experiments. Characterization of basic molecular and gene injury mechanisms that have persisted through evolution might use phylogenetically lower species such as rodents, whereas establishing the pathogenesis of impaired higher brain functions would require larger animals that have a gyrencephalic brain (one that has convolutions).

A short overview of experimental results of biologic models, mainly at the whole-animal level, provides information on mechanisms that potentially underlie long-term functional deficits or organ failure.

## Experimental Environment of Blast Generation

Experimental studies of primary blast-induced biologic responses are performed either in an open environment or in laboratory conditions. In open-field exposure studies, animals are exposed to a blast wave that is generated by detonation of an explosive (Axelsson et al., 2000; Bauman et al., 2009; Lu et al., 2012; Richmond, 1991; Saljo and Hamberger, 2004; Savic et al., 1991). Such an experimental setting is comparable with in-theater conditions, but the physical characteristics (such as homogeneity of the blast wave) are less controllable, so a broader array of biologic response should be expected.

Experiments performed in laboratory conditions use shock tubes (in which compressed air or gas generates a shock wave) or blast tubes (in which explosive charges generate a shock wave) (Nishida, 2001; Robey, 2001). The tubes focus the blast-wave energy from the source to the subject; this maximizes the blast energy (Reneer et al., 2011) without the exponential decay of the shock wave's velocity and pressure that is seen in free-field explosions (Celander et al., 1955).

The induction system routinely used in blast-exposure models consists of a cylindric metal tube divided by a plastic or metal diaphragm into two main sections: driver and driven. The anesthetized animals are fixed individually in holders that prevent movement of their bodies in response to the blast. The high pressure in the driver section is generated by an explosive charge or compressed gas and ruptures the diaphragm when it reaches the material's tolerance to pressure. After the diaphragm ruptures, the shock wave travels along the driven section with supersonic velocity and interacts with the animal. The blast overpressure duration can be varied by changing the size of the high-pressure chamber (Celander et al., 1955). The compressed atmospheric air in the tube fails to expand as quickly as would an ideal gas when the membrane is ruptured and also fails to generate a broad range of overpressure peaks. Use of a light gas, such as helium, improves the performance of the shock tubes because of the increased speed of sound in such types of gas (Celander et al., 1955; Lu and Wilson, 2003).

Although shock and blast tubes are convenient means of generating shock waves, they lack the ability to generate other factors of the blast environment, such as acoustic, thermal, optical, and electromagnetic components (Ling et al., 2009). A wide range of blast overpressure sustained for various durations has been used in single-exposure experimental studies. In most studies, the animals are subjected to a shock or blast wave that has a mean peak overpressure of 52–340 kPa (7.54–49.31 psi) on the nearest surface of an animal's body (Cernak et al., 2001b; Chavko et al., 2007; Clemedson et al., 1969; Saljo et al., 2000).

Most experiments used rodents (mice and rats) (Cernak et al., 2001a; Long et al., 2009), but some have used rabbits (Cernak et al., 1997), sheep (Savic et al., 1991), pigs (Bauman et al., 2009), or nonhuman primates (Bogo et al., 1971; Damon et al., 1968; Lu et al., 2012; Richmond et al., 1967).

## EXPERIMENTAL MODELS OF MULTIORGAN
## RESPONSES TO BLAST

### Respiratory System

*Pathologic Changes*

In the lung, damage related to spalling is exemplified by alveolar hemorrhages, whereas implosion produces air embolism from the alveoli into the pulmonary circulation (Yeh and Schecter, 2012). Blast overpressure results in primary injury to the lungs owing in part to compression of alveolar septa and capillary walls (DePalma et al., 2005). Such compression culminates in rupture of these structures, which produce interstitial edema and hemorrhage (Kirkman and Watts, 2011). The edema results in pronounced abnormal physiologic characteristics that reflect reduced gas exchange, including bradycardia, hypotension, and apnea. Brown et al. (1993) reported the first ultrastructural findings of blast lung (see Figure 3-7). They recognized the possibility that blast injury would be progres-

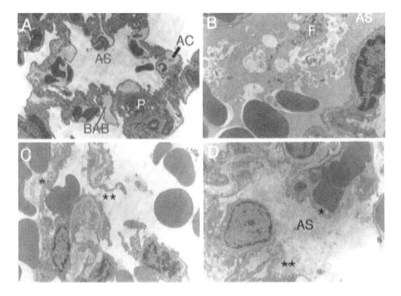

FIGURE 3-7  A. Control lung. B. Right lung 30 minutes after blast. C. Left lung 24 hours after blast. D. Right lung 24 hours after blast.
NOTES: AC = aveolar capillary; AS = alveolar space; BAB = blood–air barrier; F = fibrin clot; P = type II pneumocyte.
SOURCE: Reprinted from Brown et al. (1993). Copyright 1993, with permission from Blackwell Publishing Ltd.

sive, that is, that areas of the lung would initially appear intact but become hemorrhagic and show other signs of tissue damage. To test that, they exposed female rats to a blast wave to the right lateral surface of the lung and studied them within 30 minutes or 24 hours. Within 30 minutes, there were gross and light-microscopic distinctions between the right and left lungs. Extensive hemorrhages were restricted to the right lung. By 24 hours, however, both lungs were hemorrhagic and showed various degrees of congestion.

On electron microscopy, the *left* lung showed discrete changes in type I epithelial cells and endothelial cells by 30 minutes after the blast. The changes consisted of pinocytosis, ballooning, and rupture of the cells. The vasculature, bronchiolar epithelial cells, and related interstitium were unremarkable, and type II pneumocytes generally appeared normal in structure. These findings contrasted with those in the *right* lung, where two distinct conditions were evident 30 minutes after the blast. In the first, alveolar spaces were filled with erythrocytes, and there was little evidence of a fibrin clot. The interstitium of the alveolar walls, capillaries, and type II pneumocytes appeared intact, but there was extensive ballooning of the endothelium, and type I epithelial cells showed increased pinocytosis. The second was characterized by alveolar spaces that were filled with erythrocytes and by evidence of fibrin clotting. Alveolar walls showed interstitial disruption and capillary rupture. Intact endothelial cells exhibited ballooning, pinocytosis, and necrosis, but there was only isolated evidence of structural damage in type II pneumocytes. By 24 hours, the pathologic conditions had expanded markedly and, although the right lung was more affected than the left, both showed interstitial and intra-alveolar edema and isolated hemorrhage. Microemboli were evident in the lumina of both arterioles and venules, and the inter-alveolar septa showed more pronounced damage, with overt interstitial and intra-alveolar edema and hemorrhage. In summary, the early ultrastructural study provided confirmation that hemorrhages, present soon after blast injury, are progressive and associated with the emergence of interstitial and intra-alveolar edema, microemboli, and damage to the alveolar blood–air barrier. Collectively, those events probably compromise gas exchange and contribute to increased pulmonary vascular resistance and reduced lung compliance.

The initial study by Brown and colleagues (1993) has served as a platform for validation of blast-induced changes in the lungs in other animal models. In general, the studies reveal common pathologic features that support the earlier ultrastructural findings, namely, damage to the alveolar septa, pulmonary hemorrhage, and edema (Chavko et al., 2006; Elsayed and Gorbunov, 2007; Koliatsos et al., 2011). Koliatsos et al. (2011) confirmed the vulnerability of the lungs to blast injury and reported the following findings: intra-alveolar hemorrhages, edema, atelectasis, and inflammatory cell infiltrates. Similar findings of hemorrhages and atelectasis were reported by Zhang et al. (2011), who exposed male New Zealand rabbits to chest–abdomen blast injuries produced by explosives that were suspended above the xiphoid process. Repeated low-level blast overpressure exposures of rodents also revealed hemorrhages and ruptured alveolar walls, but the number of blast exposures did not appear to alter the magnitude of pulmonary injury; that is, the pathologic picture after repeated exposures was similar to that after a single exposure and in all cases pathologic changes increased over time (Elsayed and Gorbunov, 2007).

A proinflammatory response (that is, the activation of macrophages, lymphocytes, and neutrophils) begins within hours after blast injury. Chavko et al. (2006) evaluated inflammatory responses in male, Sprague-Dawley rats that were positioned in a shock tube and subjected to a blast wave driven by compressed air. A pronounced inflammatory response was characterized by increased expression of myeloperoxidase (MPO), an enzyme found in neutrophils, and a number of cytokines and chemokines. There is also evidence of remote damage to the lungs when blast trauma is limited to a hind limb in rodents (Ning et al., 2012). In this case, the pathologic effects over the course of 6 hours consisted of alveolar congestion and disruption, hemorrhage, and leukocyte infiltration.

### Oxidative Stress and Inflammation

Blast injury commonly results in a triad of events in the lungs (Elsayed et al., 1997): damage to structures that include the alveolar or capillary barrier and resulting hemorrhage and edema, formation of an air embolism that leads to impaired circulation and ischemia, and inflammation. Oxidative stress arises from an imbalance between oxidants and antioxidants and typically evolves as a consequence of the formation of reactive species that exceeds the capacity of antioxidant systems (see Figure 3-8). (For a more detailed review of this subject, see Elsayed and Gorbunov, 2003.) Oxidative stress may evolve as a consequence of each of those components of the triad. Pulmonary hemorrhage and the resulting accumulation of free hemoglobin trigger free-radical reactions that produce oxidative damage and support a proinflammatory state (Kirkman and Watts, 2011). Here, we address two major cascades that are triggered in part by hemorrhage and emerge within minutes to hours after injury in the lungs: oxidative stress and inflammation. Oxidative stress may lead to oxidative damage to cellular constituents, including lipids, proteins, and DNA. A number of sources may contribute to oxidative stress and injury in the lungs, including hemoglobin, which can generate reactive oxygen species (Regan and Panter, 1993), and inflammatory cells, including leukocytes and macrophages, which are key sources of reactive oxygen species (Chavko et al., 2009). Pro-oxidants

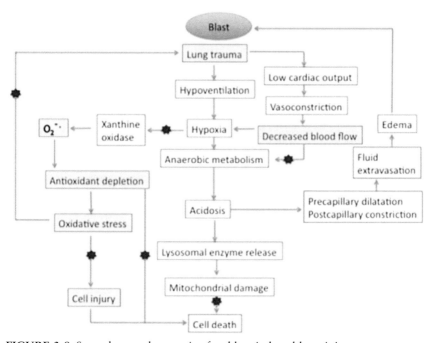

**FIGURE 3-8** Secondary pathogenesis after blast-induced lung injury.
NOTE: Red stars indicate pathways whereby antioxidants may exert protection.
SOURCE: Adapted from Elsayed and Gorbunov, 2003. Toxicology, Vol. 189, Nos.
1–2, N. M. Elsayed and N. V. Gorbunov, Interplay between high energy impulse
noise (blast) and antioxidants in the lung, pages 63–74, Copyright 2003, with
permission of Elsevier.

include both radicals (such as superoxide anion radical, hydroxyl radical, nitrogen dioxide, nitric oxides, and ethyl radicals) and nonradical reactive species (such as hydrogen peroxide, lipid hydroperoxide, hypochloric acid, and iron–oxygen complexes). Free radicals have the capacity to interact with one another to form more potent compounds, such as peroxynitrite radical resulting from the reaction of the superoxide anion radical with nitric oxide. Involvement of radicals and nonradical reactive species is complicated by the fact that although some are toxic, such as iron–oxide complexes, others may be beneficial by warding off infection or in defined contexts may act as antioxidants.

Oxidative stress and inflammation have been shown to be related key components of blast-induced damage in the lungs in a variety of experimental models (rats, rabbits, and sheep) that used low-level blast waves and blasts restricted to a limb (Chavko et al., 2006; Elsayed and Gorbunov, 2003, 2007; Gorbunov et al., 1997; Ning et al., 2012). In rats exposed to low-level blast overpressure, oxidative stress is evidenced by a 3.5-fold decrease in total antioxidant reserves and depletion of the water-soluble antioxidants ascorbate and glutathione by 50–75% and of the lipid-soluble antioxidant vitamin E by 30%. Those reductions are accompanied by lipid peroxidation and increased methemoglobin content without degradation of hemoglobin (see Table 3-3) (Gorbunov et al., 1997). Repeated low-level blast exposures result in decreases in vitamins C and E (by 20–60% and 25–40%, respectively) that are concomitant with an increase in lipid per-oxidation (by 25–50%) (Elsayed and Gorbunov, 2007). Those biochemical changes are the same whether produced by a single exposure or by multiple exposures.

Such findings suggest that repeated exposures do not compound the effects of the initial exposure. Chavko et al. (2006) evaluated the progres-sion of inflammatory and oxidative events in the lungs after exposure to medium-intensity blast overpressure. The proinflammatory response was characterized by an increase in MPO that peaked at 24 hours and increases in chemokines CINC-1 and ICAM-1 that peaked at 2–24 hours and 24–48 hours, respectively. It is thought that the early increase in CINC-1 contrib-utes to the early influx of neutrophils (MPO+). Indexes of oxidative stress (protein oxidation and nitration) and of MnSOD and heme oxygenase-1, which have antioxidative and anti-inflammatory properties, respectively, were also evaluated. Protein oxidation and nitration peaked at 2 hours. The early rise corresponded to early activation of inflammation (CINC-1) and thus implicates oxidative stress in the activation of the chemokines. Finally, the induction of MnSOD and heme oxygenase-1 at 24–48 hours after injury may not only contribute to the observed reduction in oxidative and nitrative damage that occurred later than 2 hours after injury but also facilitate the resolution of inflammation.

*Pharmacologic Manipulations of Oxidative Stress and Early Inflammation*

Pharmacologic strategies provide useful means of confirming mecha-nisms of action and establishing efficacy. N-acetylcysteine amide (NACA) and hemin, an inducer of heme oxygenase-1, are candidate therapeutics whose use has reinforced the involvement of oxidative stress and inflamma-tion in the lung after a blast. Chavko et al. (2009) evaluated NACA, focus-ing on blast-induced pulmonary inflammation. NACA is a novel derivative of N-acetylcysteine that has hydrophobic and membrane-permeable prop-erties. It has been shown to protect against hemoglobin oxidation and to reduce inflammation in a murine model of asthma (Bahat-Stroomza et al., 2005; Grinberg et al., 2005; Lee et al., 2007). Rats were given NACA 30 minutes to 24 hours after a moderate blast overpressure. It reduced infil-

**TABLE 3-3** Animal Models

| Description of Blast | Species, Sex[a] | Times Studied |
| --- | --- | --- |
| Compressed-air-driven shock tube | Sprague-Dawley rats | 5, 60 min |
| Compressed-air-driven shock tube | Sprague-Dawley rats | 1, 3, 6, 12, 24 hr |
| Compressed-air-driven shock tube | Sprague-Dawley rats | 1, 3, 6, 12, 24 hr |
| Compressed-air-driven shock tube | Sprague-Dawley rats | 15 min, 1, 3, 6, 12, 24, 34, 56 hr |
| Blast to hind limb by commercial detonator | Sprague-Dawley rats, male | 0.5, 1, 3, 6 hr |
| Compressed-air-driven shock tube | Sprague-Dawley rats, male | 1, 6, 24 hr |
| Compressed-air-driven shock tube | Sprague-Dawley rats, male | 2–192 hr |

NOTES: 3NTyr = 3-nitrotyrosine; BAL = bronchoalveolar lavage; CINC-1 = cytokine chemoattractant-1; HO-1 = heme oxygeanse-1; ICAM-1 = intercellular adhesion molecule-1; IL = interleukin; iNOS = inducible nitric oxide synthase; MCP-1 = monocyte chemoattractant protein-1; MIP-2 = macrophage inhibitory protein-2; MnSOD = manganese superoxide dismutase; MPO = myeloperoxidase; SOD = superoxide dismutase; TNF = tumor necrosis factor.
[a]Some studies do not report gender.

| Indexes of Oxidative Stress or Inflammation | Structural Changes | References |
|---|---|---|
| Decrease in total antioxidant reserves; depletion of ascorbate, glutathione, and vitamin E; increase in lipid peroxidation and methemoglobin | | Gorbunov et al., 1997 |
| In blood, decrease in iron–transferrin complexes and increase in neutrophils; in BAL fluid and blood, cytokine release (IL-1, IL-6, MCP-1, MIP-2) | | Gorbunov et al., 2005 |
| Increase in MIP-2 in plasma from 1 to 6 hr; increase in neutrophils in blood from 1 to 3 hr and decrease thereafter; no change in CD11b; transferrin-bound iron sequestration by 3 hr | Bilateral diffuse hemorrhage of alveolar septal capillaries, infiltration of neutrophils by 3 hr | Gorbunov et al., 2004 |
| Up-regulation of HO-1, MPO, 3NTyr, and SOD at 1–6 hr | Hemorrhage, deposition of hemoglobin in entire thickness of lobe; neutrophils (MPO+, CD11b+, VE-cadherin+), damage to endothelium, epithelial cell necrosis, deposition of free iron | Gorbunov et al., 2006 |
| Increase in TNF-alpha; decrease in SOD, cystathionine gamma-lyase, hydrogen sulfide | Alveolar congestion, neutrophil infiltration, hemorrhagic lesions | Ning et al., 2012 |
| Vitamins C and E decreased after initial blast by 20–60%; lipid peroxidation increased by 25–60% | After single blast, multifocal minimal to mild hemorrhage throughout lobes; by 24 hr, increased intra-alveolar hemorrhage, ruptured alveolar walls | Elsayed and Gorbunov, 2007 |
| Increases in MPO, CINC-1, ICAM-1, iNOS, protein oxidation and nitration, heme-oxygenase-1, MnSOD | | Chavko et al., 2006 |

tration of neutrophils and blocked the activation of CC chemokines, macrophage inflammatory protein-1, monocyte chemotactic peptide-1, CXC chemokine, and cytokine-induced neutrophil chemoattractant 2 and 8 days after injury. Although NACA reduced expression of heme-oxygenase-1, it had no substantial effect on MnSOD or glutathione reductase; this finding only partially supports its antioxidant effect.

Heme-oxygenase-1 is an enzyme that is responsible for the breakdown of the pro-oxidant heme to biliverdin, carbon monoxide, and ferrous iron. The free iron that is released is bound to ferritin, and this reduces its capacity to induce oxidative stress. After trauma, hemorrhage and the resulting free hemoglobin induce vasoconstriction, which results in hypoperfusion of the lung. Moreover, free iron and heme are generated from auto-oxidation of oxyhemoglobin, both of which can cause oxidative damage. Strategies to induce heme-oxygenase-1 have been shown to have therapeutic effects in different diseases. The unusual broad spectrum of its beneficial effects probably reflects its ability to function as an anti-inflammatory and cytoprotectant (via carbon monoxide) and its antioxidant properties (biliverdin and bilirubin) (Abraham and Kappas, 2005; Soares and Bach, 2009). Chavko et al. (2008) evaluated hemin, a known inducer of heme-oxygenase-1. Adult Sprague-Dawley rats were treated with hemin (treatment group) or saline (vehicle group) 20 hours before blast exposure, and euthanized 30 minutes after the blast. The blast induced heme-oxygenase-1 mRNA and protein in the lungs, but there were no differences between the treated and vehicle groups, although there was a significant difference in survival rates between the two groups: 35% survival in vehicle controls and 68% in the hemin-treated group. The authors did not speculate on the absence of differences in heme-oxygenase-1 expression between the vehicle and control (saline-treated, unexposed to blast) groups. Because the activity of the enzyme was not measured, it is conceivable that heme-oxygenase-1 activity increased in response to hemin without changes in either mRNA or protein.

### Acute Respiratory Distress Syndrome: Parallels to the Pathobiology of Blast Lung

Despite its association with a number of risk factors and inciting insults, acute respiratory distress syndrome, first described in 1967, is characterized by common mechanisms of pathogenesis as blast lung (Fanelli et al., 2013). The mechanisms include dysregulated inflammation, uncontrolled coagulation pathways, and disruption of the alveolar endothelial and epithelial barriers, which can lead to alveolar edema (Matthay et al., 2012). Leukocyte-directed proteolytic activity, oxidative stress, and excessive production of chemokines and cytokines contribute to acute lung damage. Many of those features—most notably inflammation, alveolar edema, and oxidative stress—are also signatures of blast lung. Researchers can only speculate on why that is the case. One possibility may be related to constituents of the lung that are most vulnerable to injury, namely, the alveolar endothelial and epithelial barriers that may become overwhelmed by a local proinflammatory state and the ensuing oxidative stress that results from inadequate endogenous antioxidant reserves. Considerable progress has been made in understanding the pathophysiology of acute respiratory distress syndrome. Such a foundation may prove useful to researchers who are only beginning to decipher the complex pathophysiology of blast lung and its long-term consequences.

## Abdominal Organs

The most popular explanation of primary blast-induced injuries to the abdominal organs involves the transmission of a shock wave's kinetic energy (Clemedson and Criborn, 1955) and the later generation of two main types of waves during its propagation: stress waves and shear waves. Stress waves are longitudinal pressure forces that move at supersonic speeds and create a spalling effect at the air–tissue interfaces, which results in microvascular damage and tissue disruption. Shear waves are transverse waves that cause asynchronous movement of the tissue and possible disruption at the interfaces. Stress waves cause injuries mainly to hollow organs, and shear waves, mainly to solid organs (Wightman and Gladish, 2001).

### Hollow Abdominal Organs

The most frequent primary blast-induced pathologic changes confirmed in experiments on small (Tatic et al., 1996) and large (Cripps and Cooper, 1997; Holzer et al., 2012; Savic et al., 1991) experimental animals are: widespread petechiae and localized ecchymosis in mucosa and serosa, rarely with small ulcerations. In the most severe cases, perforation of hollow gastrointestinal organs causes accumulation of air in the abdominal cavity and peritonitis. Lacerations and perforations of the diaphragm are extremely rare. Exposure to an extreme blast environment, in which primary and secondary effects act in parallel, produces immediate abdominal laceration or perforation, involving mainly the large and small bowel (Bala et al., 2008). However, contusions and intramural hematomas have been shown to predominate in nonfatal blast exposures (Cripps and Cooper, 1997); these lesions, which are morphologically and histologically similar to those caused by blunt abdominal trauma, are subject to late perforation (Cripps and Cooper, 1997; Ignjatovic et al., 1991; Paran et al., 1996). It has been suggested (Guy and Cripps, 2011) that the combined effect of stress waves and shear waves damages the mucosa and the serosa, in which the contusions at highest risk for late perforation are the ones that show evidence of subserosal bleeding rather than hemorrhage confined to the mucosa and submucosa.

Cripps and Cooper (1997) developed a blast-injury model in large white pigs that weighed 49–66 kg and had accelerometers mounted on their chests to measure the transfer of kinetic energy to the torso. Anesthetized animals were fixed to an animal holder and exposed to blast generated by detonating spherical plastic explosive charges that weighed 2.0–3.6 kg and were 1.8–3.0 m from the animal's chest wall. The animals were sacrificed after 24 hr and subjected to postmortem examination and abdominal-organ analyses. The authors provided a histologic classification of the spectrum of intestinal injury (see Table 3-4), which is consistent with injury directed from mucosa to serosa, that is, injury caused by the release of energy in the mucosa and, if energy transfer is sufficient, progressive disruption of the submucosal, muscular, and serosal layers. They concluded that serosal injury is the de facto evidence of transmural injury. Although the usual interval for perforation after blast exposure is 1–14 days, their study identified patterns of injury and a classification in which no difference was observed in the distribution of histologic grades at the two times. Thus, the authors made

**TABLE 3-4** Histologic Classification of Primary Intestinal Blast Injuries

| Grade of Injury | Mucosal Appearance | Muscular Appearance | Serosal Appearance |
|---|---|---|---|
| I[a] | Normal or diffuse bleeding only | Normal | Normal |
| II | Mucosal hematoma without glandular disruption | Mild edema only | Normal |
| III | Marked hemorrhage with glandular disruption | Marked edema or minor hemorrhage only | Normal |
| IV | Gross glandular or mucosal disruption; muscularis mucosae may be disrupted | Muscular disruption or major hematoma | Subserosal hemorrhage |
| V | Complete mucosal laceration | Muscular laceration or disruption | Serosal laceration |

[a]Includes contusions in which submucosal hematoma is evident without other evidence of mural injury.
SOURCE: Reprinted from Cripps and Cooper, 1997. Copyright 1997, with permission from Blackwell Science Ltd.

their final recommendations based on the histological features of the lesions without regard to the age of the contusion (see Table 3-5). It has been suggested that the appearance of necrosis and inflammatory cell infiltrates and the size of early pathologic changes could be predictive of perforation. If these experimental guidelines were adopted and small-bowel contusions less than 15 mm in diameter and colonic contusions smaller than 20 mm were left alone, the number of small-bowel contusions requiring excision would be reduced by one-fourth and colonic contusions by two-thirds (see Table 3-5) (Cripps and Cooper, 1997).

*Solid Organs*

Pathologic changes in solid abdominal organs (liver, spleen, pancreas, kidneys, and adrenal glands) that result from blast exposure range from subcapsular hemorrhage and small foci of parenchymal hemorrhage, to primary or secondary rupture of capsules and parenchymal laceration (Vriese, 1904). Recent experimental data clearly showed the importance of body position relative to the shock-wave front not only for injury severity but for the pattern of multi-organ damage (Koliatsos et al., 2011). Lungs, heart, and kidneys are damaged more frequently and severely when the body is supine, and the liver and spleen are injured more frequently and severely when the body is prone (see Table 3-6). In a recently published mouse blast-injury model (Koliatsos et al., 2011), liver damage was observed in a little over 40% of the cases. The pathologic changes included congestion, mottling, and white discoloration adjacent to apparently hemorrhagic sites. White infarcts were the lesion most reliably observed at the microscopic level, usually next to a distended, hemorrhaging branch of the portal vein (see Figure 3-9, panels A and B), whereas tissue ischemia was most marked around portal veins (see Figure 3-9, panel C). In contrast with lung injuries, prone position caused more severe lesions than supine position. In the prone position but not the supine position, there was some association between blast severity and infarct rate. In more severe injuries, in sheep exposed to open field blast (Savic et al., 1991; Tatic et al., 1991a; Vriese, 1904), liver laceration and subcapsular liver rupture have been reported with a lesion of the extrahepatic biliary duct and gallbladder hematoma.

The spectrum of pathologic alterations seen in pancreas, kidneys, and adrenal glands of sheep exposed to open-field blast (Savic et al., 1991; Tatic et al., 1991a; Vriese, 1904) includes petechiae, ecchymosis, and small foci of parenchymal hemorrhage. The experimental findings were comparable with findings in victims of industrial blast (Tatic et al., 1991b). In the mouse model developed by Cernak et al. (2011), the most consistent macroscopic and microscopic findings in the spleen and kidney were red infarcts. Hemorrhagic kidney infarcts occurred almost exclusively in the

62

**TABLE 3-5** Distribution of Histologic Grades Between Contusion Groups of Different External Appearance

| Contusion Measure | Histologic Grade | | | Significance | | |
|---|---|---|---|---|---|---|
| | I and II | III | IV and V | $\chi^2$ | d.f. | p |
| Size (mm) | | | | | | |
| Small bowel | | | | | | |
| ≤15 | 30 | 5 | 3 | 9.09 | 2 | 0.01 |
| >15 | 28 | 17 | 13 | | | |
| Colon | | | | | | |
| ≤20 | 60 | 4 | 3 | 14.95 | 2 | 0.0006 |
| >20 | 14 | 3 | 8 | | | |
| Position | | | | | | |
| Small bowel | | | | | | |
| Mesenteric | 18 | 12 | 11 | 7.5 | 2 | 0.02 |
| Antimesenteric | 39 | 10 | 6 | | | |
| Colon | | | | | | |
| Mesenteric | 8 | 1 | 1 | 0.12 | 2 | 0.94 |
| Antimesenteric | 66 | 6 | 10 | | | |
| Circumferential extent[a] | | | | | | |
| Small bowel | | | | | | |
| One-half or less | 47 | 13 | 6 | 14.79 | 2 | 0.0006 |
| More than one-half | 10 | 9 | 11 | | | |
| Confluence | | | | | | |
| Small bowel | | | | | | |
| Confluent | 22 | 11 | 12 | 5.49 | 2 | 0.06 |
| Diffuse | 35 | 11 | 5 | | | |
| Colon | | | | | | |
| Confluent | 26 | 4 | 8 | 6.37 | 2 | 0.04 |
| Diffuse | 48 | 3 | 3 | | | |

NOTE: d.f. = degrees of freedom.
[a]The relationship between grade and circumferential extent is not shown for the colon because only two contusions were larger than half the circumference—a feature more to do with colonic size than contusion size.
SOURCE: Reprinted from Cripps and Cooper, 1997. Copyright 1997, with permission from Blackwell Science Ltd.

TABLE 3-6 Type, Severity, and Frequency of Microscopic Lesions in Key Thoracic and Abdominal Viscera

| | Severe, Supine (%) | Severe, Prone (%) | Moderate, Supine (%) | Moderate, Prone (%) | Mild, Supine (%) | Mild, Prone (%) | Total (%)[a] |
|---|---|---|---|---|---|---|---|
| Lungs | | | | | | | |
| Superficial hemorrhages | 0.0 | 0.0 | 5.3 | 50.0 | 33.3 | 25.0 | 20.7 |
| Hematomas | 0.0 | 33.3 | 10.5 | 0.0 | 22.2 | 25.0 | 12.1 |
| Hemorrhagic consolidation | 100.0 | 66.6 | 84.2 | 50.0 | 44.4 | 37.5 | 65.5 |
| Total | | | | | | | 98.3 |
| Liver | | | | | | | |
| Infarcts | 14.3 | 100.0 | 52.6 | 50.0 | 0.0 | 50.0 | 41.4 |
| Heart | | | | | | | |
| Right ventricle dilation | 57.1 | 33.3 | 21.0 | 0.0 | 11.1 | 0.0 | 17.2 |
| Left ventricle dilation | 28.6 | 33.3 | 21.0 | 0.0 | 11.1 | 0.0 | 12.0 |
| Total | | | | | | | 29.3 |
| Spleen | | | | | | | |
| Red infarcts | 28.6 | 0.0 | 10.5 | 16.6 | 0.0 | 12.5 | 12.1 |
| Kidney | | | | | | | |
| Red infarcts | 14.3 | 0.0 | 26.3 | 8.3 | 0.0 | 0.0 | 12.1 |

[a]Percentages are rates of cases with indicated lesion out of the total number of cases in first group.
SOURCE: Reprinted with permission from Koliatsos et al., 2011 (http://links.lww.com/NEN/A233 [accessed March 27, 2014]).

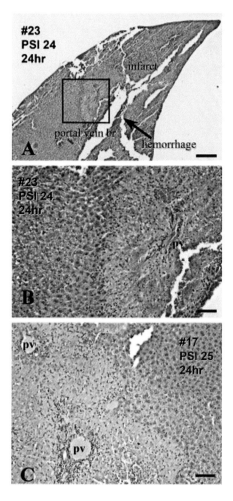

**FIGURE 3-9** Patterns of blast injury to liver with settings used in Koliatsos et al.
(2011). Hematoxylin and eosin.
NOTES: Panels A and B illustrate site of white infarct distal to a dilated or hemorrhaging branch of portal vein. Panel B is enlargement of framed area in panel A
and shows further detail of hemorrhagic smaller portal vein branch (pv) and sharp
border between normal and ischemic tissue. Panel C shows severe tissue hypoxia
around portal triads from another case. Normal liver parenchyma is shown on left
of panels A and B and right of panel C. Scale bars: A, 500 μm; B and C, 100 μm.
SOURCE: Reprinted with permission from Koliatsos et al., 2011 (http://links.lww.
com/NEN/A235 [accessed March 27, 2014]).

medullary zone (see Figure 3-10, panel A). In spleens, a dilated vessel filled with blood was seen in the trabeculae proximal to the infarct in nearly all cases (see Figure 3-10, panel B). Potential chronic consequences of blast exposure for morphologic and functional integrity of kidneys were analyzed in sheep exposed to blast (Casals et al., 2011). Substantial atrophy of parenchyma and infarction sequelae were found 30 days after exposure to a high-energy explosive-produced overpressure of 166 psi with a 3.0-ms duration (near the $LD_{50}$). It has been hypothesized that kidney contusion aided by endothelial damage of glomerular blood vessels and compromised circulation due to severed arterioles and venules may cause chronic renal insufficiency (Casals et al., 2011; Vriese, 1904). The resulting impairment

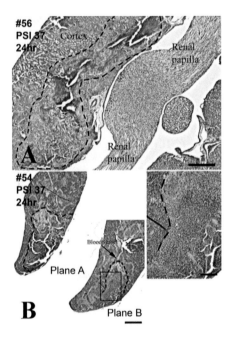

FIGURE 3-10 Pathologic signatures of blast injury to kidney (panel A) and spleen (panel B). Hematoxylin and eosin.
NOTES: A: hemorrhagic infarct in medullary zone delineated with broken line. Normal kidney parenchyma is outside broken line. B: spleen infarct associated with dilated hemorrhaging blood vessel in two planes (planes A and B). Illustration on right panel is magnification of framed area in plane B. Normal spleen parenchyma is shown on left and top. Scale bars: 500 μm.
SOURCE: Reprinted from Cernak et al., 2011, with permission from Elsevier.

of the renin–angiotensin system could lead to chronic hypertension, and this may offer a rational explanation for the hypertension noted in survivors of the Texas City explosions (Blocker and Blocker, 1949; Ruskin et al., 1948).

## Cardiovascular System

The main vascular mechanisms are described in the section on systemic changes that modify individual organ responses to blast. This section describes microvessel injury from exposure to blast in experimental models.

Zhang et al. (2011) used New Zealand rabbits exposed to explosive-generated blast in laboratory conditions to show that increased permeability, measured by $^{125}$I-albumin leakage, and microvessel injury in the lungs and kidneys are among the key outcomes of blast overpressure. Damage to the microvessels led to leakage of albumin and caused hemoconcentration in the absence of active bleeding after a blast. The resulting increase in blood viscosity and hematocrit can aggravate a blast-induced oxygen deficit and decrease vasodilation function. The microvascular endothelium is essential in maintaining circulatory homeostasis and normal physiologic function of organs. Its impairment has a broad array of implications: Diffuse microvascular hyperpermeability and later plasma extravasation may result in hypovolemic shock, pulmonary edema, abdominal compartment syndrome, and generalized tissue malperfusion (Garner et al., 2009; Lamb et al., 2010; Zhang et al., 2011).

In the mouse blast-injury model (Cernak et al., 2011), the most pronounced pathologic changes in the heart, as in the lungs, were found in animals exposed in a supine position (Koliatsos et al., 2011) (see Table 3-6). Although the animals were positioned so that their torsos were parallel to the front of the shock wave, pathologic findings were more frequent in the right side of the heart compared to the left side. The macroscopic and microscopic observations in the heart include dilation of ventricles and atria (Koliatsos et al., 2011). Venous congestion was the most frequent finding in animals exposed to mild blast, whereas dilation-filling ("congestion") of ventricles was seen with increased blast-injury severity. Hemorrhagic infarct of ventricular walls was found only in the most severe injuries. A broad array of dose-dependent pathologic changes has been reported in the hearts of sheep exposed to blast generated by detonating an aerosol bomb in an open field (Savic et al., 1991; Tatic et al., 1991a; Vriese, 1904). The findings included petechiae and ecchymosis in the pericardium, epicardium, and endocardium; hemorrhage in the myocardium; and rare endocardial hematoma.

Chronic effects of blast exposure have been demonstrated in experiments in sheep that were exposed to a high-energy explosive-produced overpressure of 164 psi with a 3.3-ms duration (near the $LD_{50}$) and sacrificed 30 days later (Casals et al., 2011). The findings included infarction sequelae in the heart in a form of multiple scars in the myocardial walls, which implied reduced cardiac contractility and compliance.

## Sensory Organs

### Fronto-Orbital Fractures

It has been posited that bone structures that provide the least resistance to transferred kinetic energy are prone to fractures when exposed to blast (Lu and Wilson, 2003). In a study that exposed 115 dogs in a shock tube to blast waves with rise times of 12–155 ms, peak overpressures of 52–231 psi, and durations of 0.4–20 s, 11 blow-out fractures (fracture of the walls or floor of the orbit) were seen in 9 animals (Guitton and Dudai, 2007). The time to and magnitude of the maximal overpressure have been shown to be critical for orbital fracture in the nearby paranasal sinuses. Orbital fractures and related eye signs have been noted in rhesus monkeys exposed to a high-explosive-produced, fast-rising overpressure of 325 psi with a duration of 3.5 ms (Casals et al., 2011). Although midface fractures in recent wars have been reported to have high complication rates (Kittle et al., 2012), there are no quantitative data that would permit an assessment of blast conditions that can be expected to produce lesions in the human orbit or make it possible to know whether the lesions are likely to be seen in survivors exposed to a combat-relevant blast environment.

### Auditory Blast

Auditory dysfunction due to blast is among the most frequent service-connected disabilities in veterans; compensation totals more than $1 billion a year (Fausti et al., 2009). Accumulating evidence demonstrates peripheral hearing loss, central auditory processing deficits, vestibular impairment, and tinnitus as the most prevalent impairments caused by blast (Fausti et al., 2009; Mehlenbacher et al., 2012; Nageris et al., 2008). The clinical manifestations of auditory blast injuries are well documented (Patterson and Hamernik, 1997), and experimental studies have provided useful information about the mechanisms underlying them.

Eardrum rupture has been posited as one of the hallmarks of blast injuries (Hirsch, 1968; White et al., 1970), but recent data indicate that the status of the tympanic membrane after exposure to a blast does not obviate further investigations to discern a primary blast injury (Peters, 2011). Early experimental data showed that tympanic membrane rupture opens the middle ear, mastoid air cells, and Eustachian tube to the invasion of pathogens and other foreign materials via the external auditory meatus. A damaged eardrum also means compromised protection of the ossicles and inner ear from overload when a single exposure to pressure variations due to blast occurs. Finally, the eardrum plays a role in energy transfer through the oval window to the organ of Corti via the ossicles and the endolymph when repetitive exposure to blast and high noise levels occurs (White et al., 1970). Using human cadavers, Zalewski (1906) demonstrated characteristic variability of the eardrum's response to overpressure that depends on age, previous scarring, calcification, infection thickening (fibrosis), unusual thinning of the tympanum, and the presence of any material in the external auditory meatus. White et al. (1970) analyzed a large series of blast experiments involving dogs, guinea pigs, goats, and rabbits and concluded that, because of the wide tolerance limits of the tympanic membrane, rupture of the eardrum or lack thereof cannot be considered a reliable clinical sign for judging the severity of a blast injury. Notably, the eardrum often remains intact when exposure pressures produce serious lung injury, but may rupture at pressures well below generally hazardous ones.

Mao et al. (2012) used a rat blast-injury model to investigate the underlying mechanisms of blast-induced tinnitus, hearing loss, and associated TBI. Briefly, anesthetized rats placed on supportive netting were subjected to a single blast exposure with a custom-designed shock tube (Leonardi et al., 2011). The 10 ms blast exposure was estimated to be in a wide range of frequencies with an average energy of under 10 kHz measured at 14 psi, which was translated to a sound pressure around 95 kPa or 194 dB above the standard reference sound pressure in air. Blast exposure induced early onset of tinnitus and central hearing impairments at a broad frequency range but showed a tendency to shift toward high frequencies over time. The immediate increase in the hearing threshold measured with auditory brainstem responses was followed by recovery on day 14; behavioral changes showed a comparable temporal profile. Diffusion-tensor magnetic resonance imaging results demonstrated substantial damage and compensatory plastic changes in some auditory brain regions; most of the changes occurred in the inferior colliculus and medial geniculate body. The authors hypothesized that the lack of important microstructural changes in the corpus callosum could be explained on the grounds that the blast exposure in their experimental setting exerted effects mainly through the auditory pathways rather than through direct impact on the brain parenchyma. Several experiments focused on mechanisms of cochlear pathology in guinea pigs (Fang, 1988; Hu, 1991; Liu, 1992a,b; Yokoi and Yanagita, 1984; Yuan, 1993; Zhai, 1991; Zhai et al., 1997), rats (Guitton and Dudai, 2007; Kirkegaard et al., 2006), and chinchillas, pigs, and sheep (Roberto et al., 1989). Effects of impulse noise exposure (25 impulses with a peak level of 165 dB SPL) on endocochlear potentials (EPs) and compound action potentials (CAPs) were investigated in guinea pigs (Fang, 1988; Zheng,

1992). The positive EPs returned to normal values 7 days after exposure but the negative EPs and the CAP threshold did not; this implied that the stria vascularis was damaged in addition to the organ of Corti. Indeed, impaired cochlear microcirculation and increased exudation of vascular stria early after impulse noise have been found by others (Kellerhals, 1972; Liu, 1992a) and suggest a potential linkage between altered microcirculation, later impaired oxygen delivery, and oxidative stress in leading to functional and morphologic impairments (Branis and Burda, 1988). A more recent study showed a smaller extent of damage to the cochlea of mice on the basis of imaging techniques newer than were used in earlier studies (Cho et al., 2013). However, although it did not show gross cochlear membrane damage, it did reveal hair-cell death and spiral ganglion neuron loss that were consistent with past studies. It has been suggested that hair-cell death could underlie chronic hearing impairments due to blast.

## Visual System

A recent mouse model of primary ocular blast injury (Hines-Beard et al., 2012) used a device that applied a localized overpressure to the eyes of experimental animals. The overpressure was generated by a device that consisted of a pressurized air tank attached to a regulated paintball gun with a machined barrel and a chamber that protected the mouse from direct injury and recoil while the eye was exposed. The experimental setting enabled analysis of the localized effects of a focused overpressure wave, but it did not reproduce a field condition in which the entire body is exposed to a blast environment. Mice were exposed to one of three blast pressures (23.6, 26.4, or 30.4 psi), and gross pathologic effects, intraocular pressure, optical coherence tomography, and visual acuity were assessed 0, 3, 7, 14, and 28 days after exposure. Focally delivered shock wave caused corneal edema, corneal abrasions, optic nerve avulsion, and retinal damage.

Clinical data demonstrated that disruption of central visual pathways represents an additional cause of blast-related visual dysfunction (Dougherty et al., 2011). In the experimental model developed by Petras et al. (1997), the effect of blast overpressure on the visual system was studied in rats exposed to blast overpressure that was generated by a compressed-air-driven shock tube. Neurologic injury to brain visual pathways was observed in male rats that survived blast overpressure exposures of 104–110 kPa and 129–173 kPa. Optic nerve fibers degenerated on the same side as the blast pressure wave. The optic chiasm contained small numbers of degenerated fibers. Optic tract fiber degeneration was present bilaterally but was predominantly on the same side. Optic tract fiber degeneration was followed to nuclear groups at the level of the midbrain, midbrain–diencephalic junction, and thalamus, where degenerated fibers arborized among the neurons of the superior colliculus, pretectal region, and lateral geniculate body. The superior colliculus contained fiber degeneration localized principally to the stratum opticum (layer III) and stratum cinereum (layer II). The pretectal area contained degenerated fibers that were widespread in the nucleus of the optic tract, olivary pretectal nucleus, anterior pretectal nucleus, and posterior pretectal nucleus. Degenerated fibers in the lateral geniculate body were not universally distributed: they appeared to arborize among neurons of the dorsal and ventral nuclei, including the ventral lateral geniculate nucleus (parvocellular and magnocellular parts) and the dorsal lateral geniculate nucleus. The study showed that blast exposure can induce permanent injury to some of the brain's central visual pathways (retinofugal axonopathy). Considering that the nuclei of the pretectal region receive connections from the superior colliculi and emit fibers to several tegmental nuclear groups implicated in coordinated movements of the eyes, the authors suggested that the blast-induced degeneration of retino-pretectal fibers might cause substantial chronic impairments in control of the pupillary light reflex and the muscles of the ciliary body for accommodation of the lens (Petras et al., 1997). Chen et al. (2003) provided further information about potential mechanisms underlying blast-induced degeneration of visual pathways. They used rabbits exposed to blast and showed that blast exposure initiates apoptosis of retinal ganglion cells parallel with increased glutamate concentration in the corpus vitreum; this suggested a potential biologic link (Chen et al., 2003).

## Heterotopic Ossification

In the recent wars in Afghanistan and Iraq, development of heterotopic ossification (HO) in residual limbs has been reported in up to 63% of people who suffered combat-related amputations (Potter et al., 2007). That was an unexpected finding in that until recent years HO has rarely been found in the residual limbs of amputees (Alfieri et al., 2012). To test the possibility that amputation of an extremity by a blast spontaneously stimulates development of HO in the residual limb, Tannous et al. (2011) developed a rat model of localized exposure of a limb to a controlled high-energy blast. The blast setup consisted of an aluminum platform placed above a water-filled steel tank. The platform contained a hole 2.5 in. in diameter and raised 1 in. above the surface of the water. A 0.75-g charge of pentaerythritol tetranitrate (PTN) was 0.5 in. beneath the surface of the water, directly beneath the center of the hole in the platform. The anesthetized rat, secured with Velcro straps onto the platform with the designated extremity positioned over the hole at the predetermined amputation level, was exposed to the kinetic energy generated by detonation of PTN submersed beneath the water surface that caused a column of water to rise at a speed of 534 m/s through the hole in the platform. The rats tolerated an isolated extremity blast injury well as long as the amputation was a forelimb amputation or a below-the-knee hind limb amputation. In this pilot experiment, three of four hindlimb amputees formed true islands of heterotopic bone in the soft tissues surrounding the amputation stump.

### Blast-Induced Neurotrauma

Blast can interact with the brain by means of (1) direct interaction with the head via direct passage of the blast wave through the skull (primary blast), which causes acceleration or rotation of the head (tertiary blast), or through the impact of particles accelerated by the energy released during the explosion (secondary blast) (Axelsson et al., 2000; Cernak et al., 1996a; Clemedson and Hultman, 1954) and (2) kinetic energy transfer of the primary blast wave to organs and organ systems, including blood in large vessels in the abdomen and chest, reaching the CNS (Irwin et al., 1999; Ohnishi et al., 2001). During the interaction with the body surface, the shock wave compresses the abdomen and chest and transfers its kinetic energy to the body's internal structures, including blood. The resulting oscillating waves traverse the body at about the speed of sound in water and deliver the shock wave's energy to the brain. Clemedson, on the basis of his extensive experimental work on shock-wave propagation through the body (Gelman, 2008; Selye, 1976; Tümer et al., 2013), was among the first scientists to suggest the possibility of shock-wave transmission to the CNS (Pang, 2001). Those two potential paths of interaction are not mutually exclusive (Rutlen et al., 1979). Most recent experimental data suggest both the importance of the blast's direct interaction with the head (Armonda et al., 2006; Axelsson et al., 2000) and the role of shock-wave-induced vascular load (Cernak et al., 1996a; Ling et al., 2009) in the pathogenesis of BINT.

Most currently used experimental models of BINT use rodents exposed to a shock wave generated in laboratory conditions with a compressed-air shock tube (Baalman et al., 2013; Cernak et al., 2011; Goldstein et al., 2012; Kamnaksh et al., 2012; Pun et al., 2011; Readnower et al., 2010; Reneer et al., 2011; Svetlov et al., 2012; Valiyaveettil et al., 2012a; Vandevord et al., 2012). Experiments with larger animals involve mainly pigs (Ahmed et al., 2012; Bauman et al., 2009) or nonhuman primates (Bogo et al., 1971; Lu et al., 2012).

Accumulating evidence suggests that primary blast causes substantial behavioral impairments and cognitive deficits in multiple animal models (Bogo et al., 1971; Cernak et al., 2001a; Lu et al., 2012). The deficits and degenerative processes in the brain show a dose–response relationship with primary blast intensity. The widely varied molecular changes start early with metabolic impairments that include altered glucose metabolism, a shift from an aerobic toward an anaerobic pathway measured as increased lactate concentration and increased lactate:pyruvate ratio (Cernak et al., 1996b), then a decline in energy reserve (Cernak et al., 1995, 1996b), development of oxidative stress (Readnower et al., 2010) in parallel with ultrastructural changes in the brainstem and hippocampus (Cernak et al., 2001b; Saljo et al., 2000) and activation of early immediate genes (Saljo et al., 2002). Later, the mechanisms include inflammation (Cernak et al., 2011; Kaur et al., 1995, 1997; Kwon et al., 2011; Readnower et al., 2010; Saljo et al., 2001), diffuse axonal injury (Garman et al., 2011; Risling et al., 2011), and apoptotic and nonapoptotic cascades that lead to neurodegeneration (Svetlov et al., 2009; Vandevord et al., 2012; Wang et al., 2010). Emerging evidence suggests that some brain structures might have a more pronounced sensitivity to blast effects either because of anatomic features and localization or because of functional properties of neuronal pathways and cells (Koliatsos et al., 2004; Valiyaveettil et al., 2012a,b). Indeed, higher sensitivity of the cerebellum and brainstem, the corticospinal system, and the optic tract has been found (Koliatsos et al., 2004) on the basis of the extent of multifocal axonal and neuronal cell degeneration. In addition, according to region-specific alterations in the activity of the enzyme acetyl-cholinesterase, the vulnerability of the frontal cortex and medulla has been observed in mice exposed to blast overpressure (Valiyaveettil et al., 2012a,b). Those changes showed a tendency toward chronicity.

The mechanisms involved in the pathobiology of BINT show some similarities with those of blunt TBI but with earlier onset of brain edema and later onset of cerebral vasospasm (see Figure 3-11) (Agoston et al., 2009). Using a pig model of blast exposure, Ahmed et al. (2012) have shown that protein biomarker concentrations in cerebrospinal fluid provide insight into the pathobiology of BINT. Their findings implicated neuronal and glial cell damage, compromised vascular permeability, and inflammation induced by blast. The early-phase biomarkers included claudin-5, vascular endothelial growth factor, and von Willebrand factor, whereas neurofilament heavy chain, neuron-specific enolase, vascular endothelial growth factor, and glial fibrillary acidic protein levels remained substantially increased compared with baseline 2 weeks after injury.

Despite the growing experimental models of BINT, there is a serious need for a well-coordinated, multidisciplinary research approach to clarify injury tolerance in animal models that are relevant to the military experience and to define the injury mechanisms that underlie acute and chronic consequences of blast exposure.

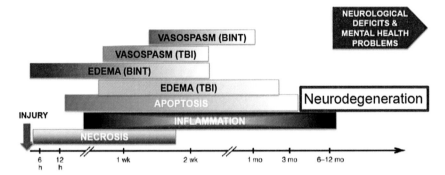

**FIGURE 3-11** Schematic representation of the approximate onset and duration of selected clinical pathologic conditions after blast TBI and nonblast TBI.
NOTE: BINT = blast-induced neurotrauma.
SOURCE: Reprinted from Agoston et al., 2009, with permission from Mary Ann Liebert, Inc. Publishers.

## REFERENCES

Abraham, N. G., and A. Kappas. 2005. Heme oxygenase and the cardiovascular-renal system. *Free Radical Biology & Medicine* 39(1):1-25

Agoston, D. V., A. Gyorgy, O. Eidelman, and H. B. Pollard. 2009. Proteomic biomarkers for blast neurotrauma: Targeting cerebral edema, inflammation, and neuronal death cascades. *Journal of Neurotrauma* 26(6):901-911.

Ahmed, F., A. Gyorgy, A. Kamnaksh, G. Ling, L. Tong, S. Parks, and D. Agoston. 2012. Time dependent changes of protein biomarker levels in the cerebrospinal fluid after blast traumatic brain injury. *Electrophoresis* 33(24):3705.

Alfieri, K. A., J. Forsberg, and B. K. Potter. 2012. Blast injuries and heterotopic ossification. *Bone and Joint Research* 1(8):192-197.

Alford, P. W., B. E. Dabiri, J. A. Goss, M. A. Hemphill, M. D. Brigham, and K. K. Parker. 2011. Blast-induced phenotypic switching in cerebral vasospasm. *Proceedings of the National Academy of Sciences of the United States of America* 108(31):12705-12710.

Armonda, R. A., R. S. Bell, A. H. Vo, G. Ling, T. J. DeGraba, B. Crandall, J. Ecklund, and W. W. Campbell. 2006. Wartime traumatic cerebral vasospasm: Recent review of combat casualties. *Neurosurgery* 59(6):1215-1225.

Axelsson, H., H. Hjelmqvist, A. Medin, J. K. Persson, and A. Suneson. 2000. Physiological changes in pigs exposed to a blast wave from a detonating high-explosive charge. *Military Medicine* 165(2):119-126.

Baalman, K. L., R. J. Cotton, S. N. Rasband, and M. N. Rasband. 2013. Blast wave exposure impairs memory and decreases axon initial segment length. *Journal of Neurotrauma* 30(9):741-751.

Bahat-Stroomza, M., Y. Gilgun-Sherki, D. Offen, H. Panet, A. Saada, N. Krool-Galron, A. Barzilai, D. Atlas, and E. Melamed. 2005. A novel thiol antioxidant that crosses the blood brain barrier protects dopaminergic neurons in experimental models of Parkinson's Disease. *European Journal of Neuroscience* 21(3):637-646.

Bala, M., A. I. Rivkind, G. Zamir, T. Hadar, I. Gertsenshtein, Y. Mintz, A. J. Pikarsky, D. Amar, N. Shussman, M. Abu Gazala, and G. Almogy. 2008. Abdominal trauma after terrorist bombing attacks exhibits a unique pattern of injury. *Annals of Surgery* 248(2):303-309.

Bass, C. R., K. A. Rafaels, and R. S. Salzar. 2008. Pulmonary injury risk assessment for short-duration blasts. *Journal of Trauma: Injury, Infection, & Critical Care* 65(3):604-615.

Bass, C. R., M. B. Panzer, K. A. Rafaels, G. Wood, J. Shridharani, and B. Capehart. 2012. Brain injuries from blast. *Annals of Biomedical Engineering* 40(1):185-202.

Bauman, R. A., G. Ling, L. Tong, A. Januszkiewicz, D. Agoston, N. Delanerolle, Y. Kim, D. Ritzel, R. Bell, J. Ecklund, R. Armonda, F. Bandak, and S. Parks. 2009. An introductory characterization of a combat-casualty-care relevant swine model of closed head injury resulting from exposure to explosive blast. *Journal of Neurotrauma* 26(6):841-860.

Ben-Dor, C., O. Igra, and T. Elperin. 2001. *Handbook of Shock Waves.* San Diego, CA: Academic Press.

Benzinger, T. 1950. Physiological effects of blast in air and water. In *German Aviation Medicine, World War II.* Volume 2. Washington, DC: Department of the Air Force. Pp. 1225-1229.

Besedovsky, H. O., and A. DelRey. 1996. Immune-neuro-endocrine interactions: Facts and hypotheses. *Endocrine Reviews* 17(1):64-102.

Blocker, V., and T. G. Blocker. 1949. The Texas City disaster: A survey of 3,000 casualties. *American Journal of Surgery* 78(5):756-771.

Bogo, V., R. A. Hutton, and A. Bruner. 1971. *The Effects of Airblast on Discriminated Avoidance Behavior in Rhesus Monkeys.* http://search.ebscohost.com/login.aspx?direct=true&db=nts&AN=AD-742+819%2fXAB&site=ehost-live (accessed October 1, 2013).

Bowen, I. G., E. R. Fletcher, D. R. Richmond, F. G. Hirsch, and C. S. White. 1968a. Biophysical mechanisms and scaling procedures applicable in assessing responses of the thorax energized by air-blast overpressures or by non-penetrating missiles. *Annals of the New York Academy of Sciences* 152(1):122-146.

Bowen, I. G., E. R. Fletcher, D. R. Richmond. 1968b. *Estimate of Man's Tolerance to the Direct Effects of Air Blast.* Washington, DC: Defense Atomic Support Agency.

Branis, M., and H. Burda. 1988. Effect of ascorbic-acid on the numerical hair cell loss in noise exposed guinea-pigs. *Hearing Research* 33(2):137-140.

Brauer, R. W., R. W. Beaver, S. Lahser, R. D. McCall, and R. Venters. 1979. Comparative physiology of the high-pressure neurological syndrome: Compression rate effects. *Journal of Applied Physiology* 46(1):128-135.

Brown, R. F., G. J. Cooper, and R. L. Maynard. 1993. The ultrastructure of rat lung following acute primary blast injury. *International Journal of Experimental Pathology* 74(2):151-162.

Casals, J. B., N. C. G. Pieri, M. L. T. Feitosa, A. C. M. Ercolin, K. C. S. Roballo, R. S. N. Barreto, F. F. Bressan, D. S. Martins, M. A. Miglino, and C. E. Ambrosio. 2011. The use of animal models for stroke research: A review. *Comparative Medicine* 61(4):305-313.

Celander, H., C. J. Clemedson, U. A. Ericsson, and H. I. Hultman. 1955. A study on the relation between the duration of a shock wave and the severity of the blast injury produced by it. *Acta Physiologica Scandinavica* 33(1):14-18.

Cernak, I. 2005. Animal models of head trauma. *NeuroRx* 2(3):410-422.

Cernak, I. 2010. The importance of systemic response in the pathobiology of blast-induced neurotrauma. *Frontiers in Neurology [electronic resource]* 1:151.

Cernak, I., and L. J. Noble-Haeusslein. 2010. Traumatic brain injury: An overview of pathobiology with emphasis on military populations. *Journal of Cerebral Blood Flow and Metabolism* 30(2):255-266.

Cernak, I., D. Ignjatovic, G. Andelic, and J. Savic. 1991. Metabolic changes as part of the general response of the body to the effect of blast waves. *Vojnosanitetski Pregled* 48(6):515-522.

Cernak, I., P. Radosevic, Z. Malicevic, and J. Savic. 1995. Experimental magnesium depletion in adult rabbits caused by blast overpressure. *Magnesium Research* 8(3):249-259.

Cernak, I., J. Savic, Z. Malicevic, D. Djurdjevic, and V. Prokic. 1996a. The pathogenesis of pulmonary blast injury: Our point of view. *Chinese Journal of Traumatology* 12(3):28-31.

Cernak, I., J. Savic, Z. Malicevic, G. Zunic, P. Radosevic, I. Ivanovic, and L. Davidovic. 1996b. Involvement of the central nervous system in the general response to pulmonary blast injury. *Journal of Trauma: Injury, Infection, & Critical Care* 40(3 Suppl):S100-S104.

Cernak, I., Z. Malicevic, and V. Prokic. 1997. Indirect neurotrauma caused by pulmonary blast injury: Development and prognosis. *International Review Armed Forces Medical Services* 52(4,5,6):114-120.

Cernak, I., J. Savic, D. Ignjatovic, and M. Jevtic. 1999a. Blast injury from explosive munitions. *Journal of Trauma: Injury, Infection, & Critical Care* 47(1):96-103; discussion 103-104.

Cernak, I., J. Savic, G. Zunic, N. Pejnovic, O. Jovanikic, and V. Stepic. 1999b. Recognizing, scoring, and predicting blast injuries. *World Journal of Surgery* 23(1):44-53.

Cernak, I., V. J. Savic, A. Lazarov, M. Joksimovic, and S. Markovic. 1999c. Neuroendocrine responses following graded traumatic brain injury in male adults. *Brain Injury* 13(12):1005-1015.

Cernak, I., Z. Wang, J. Jiang, X. Bian, and J. Savic. 2001a. Cognitive deficits following blast injury-induced neurotrauma: Possible involvement of nitric oxide. *Brain Injury* 15(7):593-612.

Cernak, I., Z. Wang, J. Jiang, X. Bian, and J. Savic. 2001b. Ultrastructural and functional characteristics of blast injury-induced neurotrauma. *Journal of Trauma: Injury, Infection, & Critical Care* 50(4):695-706.

Cernak, I., A. C. Merkle, V. E. Koliatsos, J. M. Bilik, Q. T. Luong, T. M. Mahota, L. Xu, N. Slack, D. Windle, and F. A. Ahmed. 2011. The pathobiology of blast injuries and blast-induced neurotrauma as identified using a new experimental model of injury in mice. *Neurobiology of Disease* 41(2):538-551.

Chavko, M., W. K. Prusaczyk, and R. M. McCarron. 2006. Lung injury and recovery after exposure to blast overpressure. *Journal of Trauma-Injury Infection & Critical Care* 61(4):933-942.

Chavko, M., W. A. Koller, W. K. Prusaczyk, and R. M. McCarron. 2007. Measurement of blast wave by a miniature fiber optic pressure transducer in the rat brain. *Journal of Neuroscience Methods* 159(2):277-281.

Chavko, M., W. K. Prusaczyk, and R. M. McCarron. 2008. Protection against blast-induced mortality in rats by hemin. *Journal of Trauma: Injury, Infection, & Critical Care* 65(5):1140-1145; discussion 1145.

Chavko, M., S. Adeeb, S. T. Ahlers, and R. M. McCarron. 2009. Attenuation of pulmonary inflammation after exposure to blast overpressure by n-acetylcysteine amide. *Shock* 32(3):325-331.

Chen, S., Z. Huang, L. Wang, T. Jiang, B. Wu, and G. Sun. 2003. Study on retinal ganglion cell apoptosis after explosive injury of eyeballs in rabbits. *Yen Ko Hsueh Pao [Eye Science]* 19(3):187-190.

Chiffelle, T. L. 1966. *Pathology of Direct Air-Blast Injury.* http://search.ebscohost.com/login.aspx?direct=true&db=nts&AN=AD-637+212%2fXAB&site=ehost-live (accessed October 13, 2012).

Cho, S.-I., S. S. Gao, A. Xia, R. Wang, F. T. Salles, P. D. Raphael, H. Abaya, J. Wachtel, J. Baek, D. Jacobs, M. N. Rasband, and J. S. Oghalai. 2013. Mechanisms of hearing loss after blast injury to the ear. *PLoS ONE [electronic resource]* 8(7).

Chrousos, G. P. 1995. The hypothalamine-pituitary-adrenal axis and immune-mediated inflammation. *New England Journal of Medicine* 332(20):1351-1362.

Chu, S. J., T. Y. Lee, H. C. Yan, S. H. Lin, and M. H. Li. 2005. L-arginine prevents air embolism-induced acute lung injury in rats. *Critical Care Medicine* 33(9):2056-2060.

Clemedson, C. J. 1956. Blast injury. *Physiological Reviews* 36(3):336-354.

Clemedson, C. J., and C. O. Criborn. 1955. Mechanical response of different parts of a living body to a high explosive shock wave impact. *American Journal of Physiology* 181(3):471-476.

Clemedson, C. J., and H. I. Hultman. 1954. Air embolism and the cause of death in blast injury. *Military Surgeon* 114(6):424-437.

Clemedson, C. J., and H. Pettersson. 1956. Propagation of a high explosive air shock wave through different parts of an animal body. *American Journal of Physiology* 184(1):119-126.

Clemedson, C. J., L. Frankenberg, A. Jonsson, H. Pettersson, and A. B. Sundqvist. 1969. Dynamic response of thorax and abdomen of rabbits in partial and whole-body blast exposure. *American Journal of Physiology* 216(3):615-620.

Cooper, G. J., D. J. Townend, S. R. Cater, and B. P. Pearce. 1991. The role of stress waves in thoracic visceral injury from blast loading: Modification of stress transmission by foams and high-density materials. *Journal of Biomechanics* 24(5):273-285.

Cripps, N. P., and G. J. Cooper. 1997. Risk of late perforation in intestinal contusions caused by explosive blast. *British Journal of Surgery* 84(9):1298-1303.

Damon, E. G., C. S. Gaylord, J. T. Yelverton, D. R. Richmond, I. G. Bowen, R. K. Jones, and C. S. White. 1968. Effects of ambient pressure on tolerance of mammals to air blast. *Aerospace Medicine* 39(10):1039-1047.

DePalma, R. G., D. G. Burris, H. R. Champion, and M. J. Hodgson. 2005. Blast injuries. *New England Journal of Medicine* 352(13):1335-1342.

Desmoulin, G. T., and J. P. Dionne. 2009. Blast-induced neurotrauma: Surrogate use, loading mechanisms, and cellular responses. *Journal of Trauma: Injury, Infection, & Critical Care* 67(5):1113-1122.

Dougherty, A. L., A. J. MacGregor, P. P. Han, K. J. Heltemes, and M. R. Galarneau. 2011. Visual dysfunction following blast-related traumatic brain injury from the battlefield. *Brain Injury* 25(1):8-13.

Effgen, G. B., C. D. Hue, E. Vogel, M. B. Panzer, D. F. Meaney, C. D. R. Bass, and B. Morrison. 2012. A multiscale approach to blast neurotrauma modeling. Part II: Methodology for inducing blast injury to in vitro models. *Frontiers in Neurology* 3:23.

Elsayed, N. M., and N. V. Gorbunov. 2003. Interplay between high energy impulse noise (blast) and antioxidants in the lung. *Toxicology* 189(1-2):63-74.

Elsayed, N. M., and N. V. Gorbunov. 2007. Pulmonary biochemical and histological alterations after repeated low-level blast overpressure exposures. *Toxicological Sciences* 95(1):289-296.

Elsayed, N. M., N. V. Gorbunov, and V. E. Kagan. 1997. A proposed biochemical mechanism involving hemoglobin for blast overpressure-induced injury. *Toxicology* 121(1):81-90.

Fanelli, V., A. Vlachou, S. Ghannadian, U. Simonetti, A. S. Slutsky, and H. Zhang. 2013. Acute respiratory distress syndrome: New definition, current and future therapeutic options. *Journal of Thoracic Disease* 5(3):326-334.

Fang, Y. 1988. Changes in cochlear action potential response threshold and ache in guinea pigs after blast injury. *Zhonghua Er Bi Yan Hou Ke Za Zhi* 23(6):330-333, 384.

Fausti, S. A., D. J. Wilmington, F. J. Gallun, P. J. Myers, and J. A. Henry. 2009. Auditory and vestibular dysfunction associated with blast-related traumatic brain injury. *Journal of Rehabilitation Research and Development* 46(6):797-809.

Freund, U., J. Kopolovic, and A. L. Durst. 1980. Compressed air emboli of the aorta and renal artery in blast injury. *Injury* 12(1):37-38.

Ganpule, S., A. Alai, E. Plougonven, and N. Chandra. 2012. Mechanics of blast loading on the head models in the study of traumatic brain injury using experimental and computational approaches. *Biomechanics and Modeling in Mechanobiology* 12(3):511-531.

Garman, R. H., L. W. Jenkins, R. C. Switzer, 3rd, R. A. Bauman, L. C. Tong, P. V. Swauger, S. A. Parks, D. V. Ritzel, C. E. Dixon, R. S. Clark, H. Bayir, V. Kagan, E. K. Jackson, and P. M. Kochanek. 2011. Blast exposure in rats with body shielding is characterized primarily by diffuse axonal injury. *Journal of Neurotrauma* 28(6):947-959.

Garner, J. P., S. Watts, C. Parry, J. Bird, and E. Kirkman. 2009. Development of a large animal model for investigating resuscitation after blast and hemorrhage. *World Journal of Surgery* 33(10):2194-2202.

Gelman, S. 2008. Venous function and central venous pressure: A physiologic story. *Anesthesiology* 108(4):735-748.

Goldstein, L. E., A. M. Fisher, C. A. Tagge, X. L. Zhang, L. Velisek, J. A. Sullivan, C. Upreti, J. M. Kracht, M. Ericsson, M. W. Wojnarowicz, C. J. Goletiani, G. M. Maglakelidze, N. Casey, J. A. Moncaster, O. Minaeva, R. D. Moir, C. J. Nowinski, R. A. Stern, R. C. Cantu, J. Geiling, J. K. Blusztajn, B. L. Wolozin, T. Ikezu, T. D. Stein, A. E. Budson, N. W. Kowall, D. Chargin, A. Sharon, S. Saman, G. F. Hall, W. C. Moss, R. O. Cleveland, R. E. Tanzi, P. K. Stanton, and A. C. McKee. 2012. Chronic traumatic encephalopathy in blast-exposed military veterans and a blast neurotrauma mouse model. *Science Translation Medicine* 4(134):160.

Gorbunov, N. V., N. M. Elsayed, E. R. Kisin, A. V. Kozlov, and V. E. Kagan. 1997. Air blast-induced pulmonary oxidative stress: Interplay among hemoglobin, antioxidants, and lipid peroxidation. *American Journal of Physiology* 272(2 Pt 1):L320-L334.

Gorbunov, N. V., S. J. McFaul, S. Van Albert, C. Morrissette, G. M. Zaucha, and J. Nath. 2004. Assessment of inflammatory response and sequestration of blood iron transferrin complexes in a rat model of lung injury resulting from exposure to low-frequency shock waves. *Critical Care Medicine* 32(4):1028-1034.

Gorbunov, N. V., S. J. McFaul, A. Januszkiewicz, and J. L. Atkins. 2005. Pro-inflammatory alterations and status of blood plasma iron in a model of blast-induced lung trauma. *International Journal of Immunopathology & Pharmacology* 18(3):547-556.

Gorbunov, N. V., L. V. Asher, V. Ayyagari, and J. L. Atkins. 2006. Inflammatory leukocytes and iron turnover in experimental hemorrhagic lung trauma. *Experimental & Molecular Pathology* 80(1):11-25.

Grinberg, L., E. Fibach, J. Amer, and D. Atlas. 2005. N-acetylcysteine amide, a novel cell-permeating thiol, restores cellular glutathione and protects human red blood cells from oxidative stress. *Free Radical Biology & Medicine* 38(1):136-145.

Guitton, M. J., and Y. Dudai. 2007. Blackade of cochlear NMDA receptors prevents long-term tinnitus during a brief consolidation window after acoustic trauma. *Neural Plasticity*. Published online. Article ID 80904.

Guy, R. J., and N. P. Cripps. 2011. Abdominal trauma in primary blast injury (*British Journal of Surgery* 2011; 98:168-179). *British Journal of Surgery* 98(7):1033; author reply 1033-1034.

Hines-Beard, J., J. Marchetta, S. Gordon, E. Chaum, E. E. Geisert, and T. S. Rex. 2012. A mouse model of ocular blast injury that induces closed globe anterior and posterior pole damage. *Experimental Eye Research* 99:63-70.

Hirsch, F. G. 1968. Effects of overpressure on the ear: A review. *Annals of the New York Academy of Sciences* 152(1):147-162.

Holzer, A., M. F. Pietschmann, C. Rosl, M. Hentschel, O. Betz, M. Matsuura, V. Jansson, and P. E. Muller. 2012. The interrelation of trabecular microstructural parameters of the greater tubercle measured for different species. *Journal of Orthopaedic Research* 30(3):429-434.

Hu, B. 1991. Cochlear microcirculation in living guinea pigs following explosion. *Zhonghua Er Bi Yan Hou Ke Za Zhi* 26(1):6-9, 61.

Ignjatovic, D., G. Tasic, M. Jevtic, and D. Durdevic. 1991. Occurrence and evolution of primary non-perforating lesions in blast injuries of the abdomen. *Vojnosanitetski Pregled* 48(6):523-525.

IOM (Institute of Medicine). 2009. *Gulf War and Health, Volume 7: Long-Term Consequences of Traumatic Brain Injury*. Washington, DC: The National Academies Press.

Irwin, R. J., M. R. Lerner, J. F. Bealer, P. C. Mantor, D. J. Brackett, and D. W. Tuggle. 1999. Shock after blast wave injury is caused by a vagally mediated reflex. *Journal of Trauma-Injury Infection & Critical Care* 47(1):105-110.

Kamnaksh, A., S. K. Kwon, E. Kovesdi, F. Ahmed, E. S. Barry, N. E. Grunberg, J. Long, and D. Agoston. 2012. Neurobehavioral, cellular, and molecular consequences of single and multiple mild blast exposure. *Electrophoresis* 33(24):3680-3692.

Kaur, C., J. Singh, M. K. Lim, B. L. Ng, E. P. Yap, and E. A. Ling. 1995. The response of neurons and microglia to blast injury in the rat brain. *Neuropathology & Applied Neurobiology* 21(5):369-377.

Kaur, C., J. Singh, M. K. Lim, B. L. Ng, and E. A. Ling. 1997. Macrophages/microglia as "sensors" of injury in the pineal gland of rats following a non-penetrative blast. *Neuroscience Research* 27(4):317-322.

Kellerhals, B. 1972. Acoustic trauma and cochlear microcirculation. An experimental and clinical study on pathogenesis and treatment of inner ear lesions after acute noise exposure. *Advances in Oto-Rhino-Laryngology* 18:91-168.

Khan, M. M., and K. L. Melmon. 1985. Are autocoids more than theoretic modulators of immunity? *Clinical Immunology Reviews* 4(1):1-30.

Kirkegaard, M., N. Murai, M. Risling, A. Suneson, L. Jarlebark, and M. Ulfendahl. 2006. Differential gene expression in the rat cochlea after exposure to impulse noise. *Neuroscience* 142(2):425-435.

Kirkman, E., and S. Watts. 2011. Characterization of the response to primary blast injury. *Philosophical Transactions of the Royal Society of London—Series B: Biological Sciences* 366(1562):286-290.

Kittle, C. P., A. J. Verrett, J. Wu, D. E. Mellus, R. G. Hale, and R. K. Chan. 2012. Characterization of midface fractures incurred in recent wars. *Journal of Craniofacial Surgery* 23(6):1587-1591.

Kluger, Y., A. Nimrod, P. Biderman, A. Mayo, and P. Sorkin. 2007. The quinary pattern of blast injury. *American Journal of Disaster Medicine* 2(1):21-25.

Koliatsos, V. E., T. M. Dawson, A. Kecojevic, Y. P. Zhou, Y. F. Wang, and K. X. Huang. 2004. Cortical interneurons become activated by deafferentation and instruct the apoptosis of pyramidal neurons. *Proceedings of the National Academy of Sciences of the United States of America* 101(39):14264-14269.

Koliatsos, V. E., I. Cernak, L. Xu, Y. Song, A. Savonenko, B. J. Crain, C. G. Eberhart, C. E. Frangakis, T. Melnikova, H. Kim, and D. Lee. 2011. A mouse model of blast injury to brain: Initial pathological, neuropathological, and behavioral characterization. *Journal of Neuropathology & Experimental Neurology* 70(5):399-416.

Kwon, S. K., E. Kovesdi, A. B. Gyorgy, D. Wingo, A. Kamnaksh, J. Walker, J. B. Long, and D. V. Agoston. 2011. Stress and traumatic brain injury: A behavioral, proteomics, and histological study. *Frontiers in Neurology [electronic resource]* 2:12.

Lamb, C. M., J. E. Berry, W. F. DeMello, and C. Cox. 2010. Secondary abdominal compartment syndrome after military wounding. *Journal of the Royal Army Medical Corps* 156(2):102-103.

Lee, K. S., S. R. Kim, H. S. Park, S. J. Park, K. H. Min, K. Y. Lee, Y. H. Choe, S. H. Hong, H. J. Han, Y. R. Lee, J. S. Kim, D. Atlas, and Y. C. Lee. 2007. A novel thiol compound, n-acetylcysteine amide, attenuates allergic airway disease by regulating activation of NF-kappa-B and hypoxia-inducible factor-1-alpha. *Experimental & Molecular Medicine* 39(6):756-768.

Leonardi, A. D., C. A. Bir, D. V. Ritzel, and P. J. VandeVord. 2011. Intracranial pressure increases during exposure to a shock wave. *Journal of Neurotrauma* 28(1):85-94.

Ling, G., F. Bandak, R. Armonda, G. Grant, and J. Ecklund. 2009. Explosive blast neurotrauma. *Journal of Neurotrauma* 26(6):815-825.

Liu, S. 1992a. Changes in vascular stria after blast traumatized guinea pigs by colloidal lanthanum tracing technique. *Chinese Journal of Otorhinolaryngology* 27(3):136-137, 189.

Liu, Z. 1992b. Experimental study on the mechanism of free radical in blast trauma induced hearing loss. *Chinese Journal of Otorhinolaryngology* 27(1):24-26, 61.

Long, J. B., T. L. Bentley, K. A. Wessner, C. Cerone, S. Sweeney, and R. A. Bauman. 2009. Blast overpressure in rats: Recreating a battlefield injury in the laboratory. *Journal of Neurotrauma* 26(6):827-840.

Lu, F. K., and D. R. Wilson. 2003. Detonation driver for enhancing shock tube performance. *Shock Waves* 12(6):457-468.

Lu, J., K. C. Ng, G. Ling, J. Wu, D. J. Poon, E. M. Kan, M. H. Tan, Y. J. Wu, P. Li, S. Moochhala, E. Yap, L. K. Lee, M. Teo, I. B. Yeh, D. M. Sergio, F. Chua, S. D. Kumar, and E. A. Ling. 2012. Effect of blast exposure on the brain structure and cognition in macaca fascicularis. *Journal of Neurotrauma* 29(7):1434-1454.

Magnuson, J., F. Leonessa, and G. S. F. Ling. 2012. Neuropathology of explosive blast traumatic brain injury. *Current Neurology and Neuroscience Reports* 1-10.

Mainiero, R., and M. Sapko. 1996. *Blast and Fire Propagation in Underground Facilities.* Technical report no. DNA-TR-93-159. Alexandria, VA: Defense Nuclear Agency.

Mao, J. C., E. Pace, P. Pierozynski, Z. Kou, Y. Shen, P. Vandevord, E. M. Haacke, X. Zhang, and J. Zhang. 2012. Blast-induced tinnitus and hearing loss in rats: Behavioral and imaging assays. *Journal of Neurotrauma* 29(2):430-444.

Mason, W. v. H., T. G. Damon, A. R. Dickinson, and T. O. Nevison, Jr. 1971. Arterial gas emboli after blast injury. *Proceedings of the Society for Experimental Biology & Medicine* 136(4):1253-1255.

Matthay, M. A., L. B. Ware, and G. A. Zimmerman. 2012. The acute respiratory distress syndrome. *Journal of Clinical Investigation* 122(8):2731-2740.

Mayorga, M. A. 1997. The pathology of primary blast overpressure injury. *Toxicology* 121(1):17-28.

Mehlenbacher, A., B. Capehart, D. Bass, and J. R. Burke. 2012. Sound induced vertigo: Superior canal dehiscence resulting from blast exposure. *Archives of Physical Medicine & Rehabilitation* 93(4):723-724.

Mellor, S. G. 1988. The pathogenesis of blast injury and its management. *British Journal of Hospital Medicine* 39(6):536-539.

Melmon, K. L., R. E. Rocklin, and R. P. Rosenkranz. 1981. Autacoids as modulators of the inflammatory and immune response. *American Journal of Medicine* 71(1):100-106.

Moss, W. C., M. J. King, and E. G. Blackman. 2009. Skull flexure from blast waves: A mechanism for brain injury with implications for helmet design. *Physical Review Letters* 103(10):108702.

Nageris, B. I., J. Attias, and R. Shemesh. 2008. Otologic and audiologic lesions due to blast injury. *Journal of Basic & Clinical Physiology & Pharmacology* 19(3-4):185-191.

Nevison, T. O., Jr., W. V. Mason, and A. R. Dickinson. 1971. *Measurement of blood velocity and detection of emboli by ultrasonic doppler technique.* Paper presented at 11th Annual Symposium on Experimental Mechanics, Albuquerque, NM.

Ning, J. L., L. W. Mo, K. Z. Lu, X. N. Lai, Z. G. Wang, and D. Ma. 2012. Lung injury following lower extremity blast trauma in rats. *Journal of Trauma and Acute Care Surgery* 73(6):1537-1544.

Nishida, M. 2001. Shock tubes and tunnels: Facilities, instrumentation, and techniques. Shock tubes. In *Handbook of Shock Waves,* edited by C. Ben-Dor, O. Igra, and T. Elperin. San Diego: Academic Press. Pp. 553-585.

Ohnishi, M., E. Kirkman, R. J. Guy, and P. E. Watkins. 2001. Reflex nature of the cardiorespiratory response to primary thoracic blast injury in the anaesthetised rat. *Experimental Physiology* 86(3):357-364.

Owen-Smith, M. S. 1981. Hunterian lecture 1980: A computerized data retrieval system for the wounds for war: The Northern Ireland casualties. *Journal of the Royal Army Medical Corps* 127(1):31-54.

Paintal, A. S. 1969. Mechanism of stimulation of type J pulmonary receptors. *Journal of Physiology—London* 203(3):511.

Pang, C. C. Y. 2001. Autonomic control of the venous system in health and disease: Effects of drugs. *Pharmacology & Therapeutics* 90(2-3):179-230.

Panzer, M. B., K. A. Matthews, A. W. Yu, B. Morrison, 3rd, D. F. Meaney, and C. R. Bass. 2012. A multiscale approach to blast neurotrauma modeling. Part I: Development of novel test devices for in vivo and in vitro blast injury models. *Frontiers in Neurology [electronic resource]* 3:46.

Paran, H., D. Neufeld, I. Shwartz, D. Kidron, S. Susmallian, A. Mayo, K. Dayan, I. Vider, G. Sivak, and U. Freund. 1996. Perforation of the terminal ileum induced by blast injury: Delayed diagnosis or delayed perforation? *Journal of Trauma: Injury, Infection, & Critical Care* 40(3):472-475.

Patterson, J. H., Jr., and R. P. Hamernik. 1997. Blast overpressure induced structural and functional changes in the auditory system. *Toxicology* 121(1):29-40.

Peters, P. 2011. Primary blast injury: An intact tympanic membrane does not indicate the lack of a pulmonary blast injury. *Military Medicine* 176(1):110-114.

Petras, J. M., R. A. Bauman, and N. M. Elsayed. 1997. Visual system degeneration induced by blast overpressure. *Toxicology* 121(1):41-49.

Phillips, Y. Y. 1986. Primary blast injuries. *Annals of Emergency Medicine* 15(12):1446-1450.

Potter, B. K., T. C. Burns, A. P. Lacap, R. R. Granville, and D. A. Gajewski. 2007. Heterotopic ossification following traumatic and combat-related amputations. Prevalence, risk factors, and preliminary results of excision. *Journal of Bone & Joint Surgery—American Volume* 89(3):476-486.

Pun, P. B., E. M. Kan, A. Salim, Z. Li, K. C. Ng, S. M. Moochhala, E. A. Ling, M. H. Tan, and J. Lu. 2011. Low level primary blast injury in rodent brain. *Frontiers in Neurology [electronic resource]* 2:19.

Readnower, R. D., M. Chavko, S. Adeeb, M. D. Conroy, J. R. Pauly, R. M. McCarron, and P. G. Sullivan. 2010. Increase in blood-brain barrier permeability, oxidative stress, and activated microglia in a rat model of blast-induced traumatic brain injury. *Journal of Neuroscience Research* 88(16):3530-3539.

Regan, R. F., and S. S. Panter. 1993. Neurotoxicity of hemoglobin in cortical cell culture. *Neuroscience Letters* 153(2):219-222.

Reneer, D. V., R. D. Hisel, J. M. Hoffman, R. J. Kryscio, B. T. Lusk, and J. W. Geddes. 2011. A multi-mode shock tube for investigation of blast-induced traumatic brain injury. *Journal of Neurotrauma* 28(1):95-104.

Rice, D., and J. Heck. 2000. Terrorist bombings: Ballistics, patterns of blast injury and tactical emergency care. *Tactical Edge Journal* Summer:53-55.

Richmond, D. R. 1991. Blast criteria for open spaces and enclosures. *Scandinavian Audiology Supplementum* 34:49-76.

Richmond, D. R., E. G. Damon, I. G. Bowen, E. R. Fletcher, and C. S. White. 1967. Air-blast studies with eight species of mammals. Technical progress report DASA 1854. *Fission Product Inhalation Project* 1-44.

Richmond, D. R., E. G. Damon, E. R. Fletcher, I. G. Bowen, and C. S. White. 1968. The relationship between selected blast-wave parameters and the response of mammals exposed to air blast. *Annals of the New York Academy of Sciences* 152(1):103-121.

Risling, M., and J. Davidsson. 2012. Experimental animal models for studies on the mechanisms of blast-induced neurotrauma. *Frontiers in Neurology [electronic resource]* 3:30.

Risling, M., S. Plantman, M. Angeria, E. Rostami, B. M. Bellander, M. Kirkegaard, U. Arborelius, and J. Davidsson. 2011. Mechanisms of blast induced brain injuries, experimental studies in rats. *Neuroimage* 54(Suppl 1):S89-S97.

Roberto, M., R. P. Hamernik, and G. A. Turrentine. 1989. Damage of the auditory system associated with acute blast trauma. *Annals of Otology, Rhinology, & Laryngology—Supplement* 140:23-34.

Roberts, J. C., T. P. Harrigan, E. E. Ward, T. M. Taylor, M. S. Annett, and A. C. Merkle. 2012. Human head-neck computational model for assessing blast injury. *Journal of Biomechanics* 45(16):2899-2906.

Robey, R. 2001. Shock tubes and tunnels: Facilities, instrumentation, and techniques. Blast tubes. In *Handbook of Shock Waves*, edited by C. Ben-Dor, O. Igra, and T. Elperin. San Diego: Academic Press. Pp. 623-650.

Rossle, R. 1950. Pathology of blast effects. In *German Aviation Medicine, World War II, Volume 2*. Washington, DC: Department of the Air Force.

Ruskin, A., O. W. Beard, and R. L. Schaffer. 1948. Blast hypertension: Elevated arterial pressures in the victims of the Texas City disaster. *American Journal of Medicine* 4(2):228-236.

Rutlen, D. L., E. W. Supple, and W. J. Powell. 1979. Role of the liver in the adrenergic regulation of blood-flow from the splanchnic to the central circulation. *Yale Journal of Biology and Medicine* 52(1):99-106.

Saljo, A., and A. Hamberger. 2004. *Intracranial sound pressure levels during impulse noise exposure*. Paper presented at 7th International Neurotrauma Symposium, Adelaide, Australia.

Saljo, A., F. Bao, K. G. Haglid, and H. A. Hansson. 2000. Blast exposure causes redistribution of phosphorylated neurofilament subunits in neurons of the adult rat brain. *Journal of Neurotrauma* 17(8):719-726.

Saljo, A., F. Bao, and A. Hamberger. 2001. Exposure to short-lasting impulse noise causes microglial and astroglial cell activation in the adult rat brain. *Pathophysiology* 8(2):105-111.

Saljo, A., F. Bao, J. S. Shi, A. Hamberger, H. A. Hansson, and K. G. Haglid. 2002. Expression of c-fos and c-myc and deposition of beta-app in neurons in the adult rat brain as a result of exposure to short-lasting impulse noise. *Journal of Neurotrauma* 19(3):379-385.

Savic, J., V. Tatic, D. Ignjatovic, V. Mrda, D. Erdeljan, I. Cernak, S. Vujnov, M. Simovic, G. Andelic, and M. Duknic. 1991. Pathophysiologic reactions in sheep to blast waves from detonation of aerosol explosives. *Vojnosanitetski Pregled* 48(6):499-506.

Selye, H. 1976. 40 years of stress research: Principal remaining problems and misconceptions. *Canadian Medical Association Journal* 115(1):53-56.

Soares, M. P., and F. H. Bach. 2009. Heme oxygenase-1: From biology to therapeutic potential. *Trends in Molecular Medicine* 15(2):50-58.

Stewart, C. 2014. Blast injuries: True weapons of mass destruction. www.storysmith.net/page7/page15/files/page15_5.doc (accessed January, 14, 2014).

Surbatovic, M., N. Filipovic, S. Radakovic, N. Stankovic, and Z. Slavkovic. 2007. Immune cytokine response in combat casualties: Blast or explosive trauma with or without secondary sepsis. *Military Medicine* 172(2):190-195.

Svetlov, S., V. Prima, D. Kirk, J. Atkinson, H. Gutierrez, K. Curley, R. Hayes, and K. Wang. 2009. Morphological and biochemical signatures of brain injury following head-directed controlled blast overpressure impact. *Journal of Neurotrauma* 26(8):A75.

Svetlov, S. I., V. Prima, O. Glushakova, A. Svetlov, D. R. Kirk, H. Gutierrez, V. L. Serebruany, K. C. Curley, K. K. W. Wang, and R. L. Hayes. 2012. Neuro-glial and systemic mechanisms of pathological responses in rat models of primary blast overpressure compared to "composite" blast. *Frontiers in Neurology [electronic resource]* 3:15.

Tannous, O., C. Griffith, R. V. O'Toole, and V. D. Pellegrini, Jr. 2011. Heterotopic ossification after extremity blast amputation in a Sprague-Dawley rat animal model. *Journal of Orthopaedic Trauma* 25(8):506-510.

Tatic, V., D. Ignjatovic, V. Mrda, and J. Savic. 1991a. Morphologic changes in the tissues and organs of sheep in blast injuries caused by detonation of aerosol explosives. *Vojnosanitetski Pregled* 48(6):541-545.

Tatic, V., Z. Stankovic, and Z. Hadzic. 1991b. Morphologic damage in internal organs in miners caused by explosions of methane gas in mines. *Vojnosanitetski Pregled* 48(6):547-550.

Tatic, V., D. Ignjatovic, M. Jevtic, M. Jovanovic, M. Draskovic, and D. Durdevic. 1996. Morphologic characteristics of primary nonperforative intestinal blast injuries in rats and their evolution to secondary perforations. *Journal of Trauma: Injury, Infection, & Critical Care* 40(3 Suppl):S94-S99.

Tsokos, M., F. Paulsen, S. Petri, B. Madea, K. Puschel, and E. E. Turk. 2003a. Histologic, immunohistochemical, and ultrastructural findings in human blast lung injury. *American Journal of Respiratory & Critical Care Medicine* 168(5):549-555.

Tsokos, M., E. E. Turk, B. Madea, E. Koops, F. Longauer, M. Szabo, W. Huckenbeck, P. Gabriel, and J. Barz. 2003b. Pathologic features of suicidal deaths caused by explosives. *American Journal of Forensic Medicine & Pathology* 24(1):55-63.

Tümer, N., S. Svetlov, M. Whidden, N. Kirichenko, V. Prima, B. Erdos, A. Sherman, F. Kobeissy, R. Yezierski, P. J. Scarpace, C. Vierck, and K. K. W. Wang. 2013. Overpressure blast-wave induced brain injury elevates oxidative stress in the hypothalamus and catecholamine biosynthesis in the rat adrenal medulla. *Neuroscience Letters* 544:62-67.

Valiyaveettil, M., Y. Alamneh, S. Oguntayo, Y. Wei, Y. Wang, P. Arun, and M. P. Nambiar. 2012a. Regional specific alterations in brain acetylcholinesterase activity after repeated blast exposures in mice. *Neuroscience Letters* 506(1):141-145

Valiyaveettil, M., Y. A. Alamneh, S. A. Miller, R. Hammamieh, P. Arun, Y. Wang, Y. Wei, S. Oguntayo, J. B. Long, and M. P. Nambiar. 2012b. Modulation of cholinergic pathways and inflammatory mediators in blast-induced traumatic brain injury. *Chemico-Biological Interactions* 203(1):371-375.

Valiyaveettil, M., Y. Alamneh, Y. Wang, P. Arun, S. Oguntayo, Y. Wei, J. B. Long, and M. P. Nambiar. 2013. Contribution of systemic factors in the pathophysiology of repeated blast-induced neurotrauma. *Neuroscience Letters* 539:1-6.

Vandevord, P. J., R. Bolander, V. S. Sajja, K. Hay, and C. A. Bir. 2012. Mild neurotrauma indicates a range-specific pressure response to low level shock wave exposure. *Annals of Biomedical Engineering* 40(1):227-236.

Vriese, B. 1904. Sur la signification morfologique des artères céfebrales. *Archives de Biologie (Liege)* 21:357-457.

Wang, Y., Z. Ye, X. Hu, J. Huang, and Z. Luo. 2010. Morphological changes of the neural cells after blast injury of spinal cord and neuroprotective effects of sodium beta-aescinate in rabbits. *Injury* 41(7):707-716.

White, C. S., I. G. Bowen, and D. R. Richmond. 1965. Biological tolerance to air blast and related biomedical criteria. Cex-65.4. *Cex Reports, Civil Effects Exercise* 1-239.

White, C. S., I. G. Bowen, and D. R. Richmond. 1970. The relation between eardrum failure and blast induced pressure variations. *Space Life Sciences* 2(2):158-205

Wightman, J. M., and S. L. Gladish. 2001. Explosions and blast injuries. *Annals of Emergency Medicine* 37(6):664-678.

Wilkinson, C. W., K. F. Pagulayan, E. C. Petrie, C. L. Mayer, E. A. Colasurdo, J. B. Shofer, K. L. Hart, D. Hoff, M. A. Tarabochia, and E. R. Peskind. 2012. High prevalence of chronic pituitary and target-organ hormone abnormalities after blast-related mild traumatic brain injury. *Frontiers in Neurology* 3:11.

Yeh, D. D., and W. P. Schecter. 2012. Primary blast injuries: An updated concise review. *World Journal of Surgery* 36(5):966-972.

Yokoi, H., and N. Yanagita. 1984. Blast injury to sensory hairs: A study in the guinea pig using scanning electron microscopy. *Archives of Oto-Rhino-Laryngology* 240(3):263-270.

Yuan, Y. G. 1993. Relationship between intracochlear oxygen tension and acoustic trauma following explosion. *Chinese Journal of Otorhinolaryngology* 28(4):222-224, 252.

Zalewski, T. 1906. Experimentelle untersuchungen uber die resistensfahigkeit des trommelells. *Z Ohrenheilklinik* 52:109-128.

Zhai, S. 1991. Effects of explosions on cortical response threshold and enzyme activities in inner ear of guinea pigs. *Chinese Journal of Otorhinolaryngology* 26(2):73-75, 124.

Zhai, S., J. Cheng, and J. Wang. 1997. Treatment effects of fibroblast growth factors on blast-induced hearing loss. *Chinese Journal of Otorhinolaryngology* 32(6):354-356.

Zhang, B., A. Wang, W. Hu, L. Zhang, Y. Xiong, J. Chen, and J. Wang. 2011. Hemoconcentration caused by microvascular dysfunction after blast injuries to the chest and abdomen of rabbits. *Journal of Trauma-Injury Infection & Critical Care* 71(3):694-701.

Zheng, J. F. 1992. Effect of impulse noise exposure on the endocochlear potentials. *Zhonghua Er Bi Yan Hou Ke Za Zhi* 27(6):328-330, 381.

Zucker, I. H. 1986. Left-ventricular receptors: Physiological controllers or pathological curiosities. *Basic Research in Cardiology* 81(6):539-557.

Zuckerman, S. 1940. Experimental study of blast injuries to the lung. *Lancet* 2:219-224.

# 4

# Human Health Outcomes

Explosive blasts can cause multiple forms of damage that are more complex than those caused by other wounding agents (Champion et al., 2009). Blasts are the leading cause of death and injury on the military battlefield (Eastridge et al., 2012). Recent reports indicate that almost 80% of all combat-related injuries in US military personnel deployed to Iraq and Afghanistan have been from blasts; this is the highest proportion seen in any large-scale conflict (Murray et al., 2005; Owens et al., 2008). During the last decade, the incidence of primary blast injury and injury severity increased, and return-to-duty rates decreased. Despite increased injury severity, mortality due to explosion injuries remained low and unchanged (Kelly et al., 2008; Ritenour et al., 2010). The acute physical and psychologic human health outcomes in those who survive blast explosions can be devastating. The long-term consequences are less clear.

This chapter summarizes the committee's evaluation of the literature on the association between exposure to blast and short- and long-term effects on the human body. The guidelines agreed on by the committee and used to determine which studies to include in the evidence review below are described in Chapter 2. The chapter is organized by health outcomes: psychologic and psychiatric, nervous system, auditory and vestibular, ocular, cardiovascular, respiratory, digestive system, genitourinary (GU), dermal, and musculoskeletal outcomes; infections; and burns. The organization generally follows that of the *International Classification of Diseases, Ninth Revision*. The final section, on blast protection, evaluates whether improvements in blast protection are associated with diminished blast injury.

Although the information here is presented by individual organ systems

**Acute blast: Vulnerable**                    **Long-term**
**organs/systems**                         **Secondary Effects**

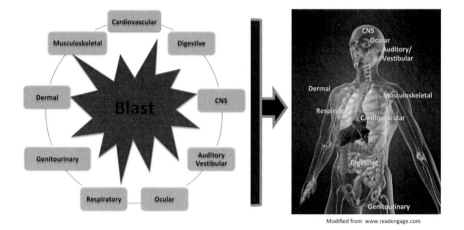

Modified from  www.readengage.com

FIGURE 4-1 Blast injury may result in primary damage to a number of organ systems. Less studied are the effects that primary damage to a specified organ may have on the long-term consequences of the functioning of other organs. For example, exposure to a blast may result in air emboli that develop from damaged lungs at alveolar–pulmonary venous fistulae and cause myocardial ischemia or infarction and thus compromise long-term cardiac function. Damage to the brain may result in motor weakness; voiding dysfunction, such as an overactive (spastic) or, over time, hypoactive bladder; change in auditory processing abilities; visual symptoms; and hypogonadism caused by hypopituitarism. Damage to the cardiovascular system can affect neurologic function through ischemia, which, if sufficiently severe, can lead to permanent brain damage.
SOURCE: Created by Linda Noble-Haeusslein for the Committee on Gulf War and Health: Long-Term Effects of Blast Exposures; figure of the human body adapted from www.readengage.com.

and specific outcomes, exposure to blast often leads to polytrauma (that is, multiple traumatic injuries) and results in a multisystem response. The section of Chapter 3 titled "Modifying Potential of Systemic Changes Caused by Blast" describes how the complexity of the blast environment can lead to changes in systemic, local, and cerebral responses. Four important systemic alterations—air emboli, activation of the autonomic nervous system, vascular mechanisms, and systemic inflammation—are explained in detail there.

Figure 4-1 illustrates how damage to an organ from exposure to blast may have long-term consequences for the functioning of other organs.

Nearly all of the epidemiologic studies evaluated by the committee relied on self-reported exposure to blast, not objective measures. The mechanism of blast—primary, secondary, tertiary, quaternary, or quinary—generally was not reported in the studies. As detailed in the committee's recommendations in Chapter 5, obtaining accurate, objective measurement of exposure to blast is essential for understanding the mechanisms of injury caused by blast.

## PSYCHOLOGIC AND PSYCHIATRIC OUTCOMES

The potential relationship between blast and its psychologic and psychiatric outcomes is different from the relationships with other organ systems reviewed. Currently, it is not known whether the primary blast wave itself results in any direct physiologic or neuroanatomic changes to the nervous system that cause acute or long-term mental disorders. That knowledge is in contrast with other etiologies of traumatic brain injury (TBI) in which there is physical evidence of neurotrauma (Bazarian et al., 2013; Jorge et al., 2012). However, blast explosions often result in tremendous human carnage in the form of severe, mutilating injuries and death. During the immediate aftermath of blasts (sometimes referred to as the aftermath of battle [Stein et al., 2012]), people often remember the carnage, which can haunt them for days, months, or years. Blast explosions, such as those caused by improvised explosive devices, have been the greatest cause of death and injury in US military personnel deployed to Iraq and Afghanistan (Champion et al., 2009; Ritenour et al., 2010), and exposure to the aftermath of blasts during deployment is probably an important cause of acute and long-term psychologic and psychiatric disorders in military service members and veterans. Whether the relationship between blasts and health outcomes is primary (in which an injury is caused directly by the blast wave itself) or secondary (in which an injury is a reaction to the emotional impact of the blast) is debatable. According to the *Diagnostic and Statistical Manual of Mental Disorders* (APA, 2013), witnessing the devastation of a blast explosion would be considered exposure to primary trauma. For the purpose of the present review, blast was evaluated as a primary cause of behavioral health outcomes, even though in some instances it is the psychologic impact and interpretation of the aftermath of a blast that potentially result in a psychologic injury rather than the direct physical impact of the blast wave itself.

## Acute Effects

Exposure to blast has a number of acute psychologic and psychiatric outcomes. Distress reactions that occur within the first 3 days after a blast exposure are considered normal and are referred to as acute stress reactions (WHO, 2010). Acute stress reactions are transient disorders in which symptoms develop within minutes of exposure to a traumatic event. The symptoms usually subside within hours or days with resumption of routine activities, when possible, and general support from friends, family, or co-workers. In most cases, professional intervention is not required.

When the signs and symptoms of acute stress reactions cluster and arrange in specific combinations and last for at least 3 days, they can lead to a diagnosis of acute stress disorder (APA, 2013). Acute stress disorder includes symptoms of intrusion, negative mood, dissociation, avoidance, and hyperarousal. The symptoms last from 3 days to a month after the trauma exposure. If they persist for more than 1 month, the diagnosis of posttraumatic stress disorder (PTSD) should be considered (APA, 2013).

Adjustment disorders are other possible acute outcomes of blast exposure in people who do not meet diagnostic criteria for acute stress disorder (APA, 2013). Adjustment disorders include the development of emotional and behavioral symptoms in response to an identifiable stressor, such as a blast, that occurs within 3 months after the event. Major depressive disorder may also be diagnosed using a separate cluster of the same symptoms at 2 weeks' duration (APA, 2013).

Regardless of whether a person meets the diagnostic criteria for these acute outcomes, it is often only when the symptoms persist over an extended period that most psychologic and psychiatric disorders are identified.

## Long-Term Effects

PTSD is the primary long-term sequela of combat-related trauma exposure, such as that experienced as a result of blasts (Peterson et al., 2011; Tanielian and Jaycox, 2008). Few studies have directly evaluated the long-term psychologic and psychiatric outcomes (for example, major depressive disorder, substance-abuse disorders, postconcussive syndrome [related to TBI], sleep disorders, marital and family discord, and suicide) of blast exposure beyond PTSD. Therefore, the present review focuses on PTSD. The long-term effects of TBI from blast are reviewed in the later section "Nervous System Outcomes."

The lifetime prevalence of PTSD has been reported to be 8.0% in the adult US population (4.0% in males and 11.7% in females) (Kessler et al., 2012). Sex differences in population surveys are related primarily to differences in frequency and type of trauma exposure. Females are more likely to be victims of sexual assault, and males are more likely to experience combat-related trauma (Kessler et al., 1995, 2005). However, when trauma type and frequency are controlled for, sex differences in PTSD are less likely to be found. For example, in a large sample of UK armed forces personnel, men (5.0%) and women (4.2%) reported similar rates of PTSD symptoms after deployment to Iraq (Rona et al., 2007). Similarly, US military men (2.3%) and women (2.3%) experienced the same rates of PTSD symptoms after serving in the war in Iraq (DOD, 2007). Such findings have led some to conclude that the risk of PTSD in military personnel "has more to do with the intensity and frequency of combat experience than gender" (Hoge et al., 2007, p. 328).

To evaluate the long-term psychiatric and psychologic health effects of blast exposure, the committee reviewed 40 relevant published peer-reviewed studies that involved some measure of blast injury. Only two met enough of the inclusion guidelines to be considered primary (see Table 4-1) (Bazarian et al., 2013; Polusny et al., 2011). This section details the primary studies and supportive studies of long-term psychiatric and psychologic health outcomes of blast exposure.

### Primary Studies

Polusny et al. (2011) conducted a longitudinal cohort study of combat-deployed National Guard members to assess the associations between mild TBI and PTSD symptoms reported in theater and longer-term psychosocial outcomes. Participants in the study were surveyed in Iraq a month before redeploying home (time 1, during redeployment transition briefings held at military installations in the Iraq combat theater) and again a year later (time 2, with mailed surveys). The first survey included 2,677 National Guard members, and 953 completed the followup survey at time 2. The surveys incorporated the following screening tools to gather outcome measures: the PTSD Checklist–Military, the Beck Depression Inventory, the Patient Health Questionnaire, the Alcohol Use Disorders Identification Test (AUDIT), World Health Organization Quality of Life–Brief, and self-reports of blast-related mild TBI, which was defined as an injury during deployment with loss of consciousness or altered mental status.

Of the 953 participants surveyed at time 2, 206 (22%) reported having a blast injury. Results for self-reported mild TBI during deployment showed 9.2% at time 1 and 22.0% at time 2. Service members who had a history of mild TBI were more likely than those who did not to report post-deployment postconcussive symptoms and poorer psychosocial outcomes. However, after adjustment for self-reported PTSD symptoms, mild TBI was not associated with post-deployment symptoms or outcomes. Time 1 PTSD symptoms predicted postdeployment PTSD and mild TBI symptoms and

TABLE 4-1 Psychiatric and Postconcussive Symptoms—Primary Studies

| Reference | Study Design | Population | Health Outcomes or Outcome Measures |
|---|---|---|---|
| Bazarian et al., 2013 | Nested cohort | Parent cohort consisted of 500 OEF or OIF veterans; subset examined in study included 52 OEF or OIF combat veterans assessed 4 years after last tour of duty | Self-report of blast exposure and TBI symptoms, PTSD Checklist–Military, combat experiences survey, anatomical MRI, DTI |
| Polusny et al., 2011 | Longitudinal cohort | 953 US National Guard brigade combat team assessed in Iraq 1 month before return (time 1) and 1 year later (time 2) | Self-report concussion or mild TBI defined as an injury during deployment with loss of consciousness (LOC) or altered mental status; PTSD checklist–military; Beck Depression Inventory; Patient Health Questionnaire (somatic symptoms); postconcussive symptoms, AUDIT (alcohol); WHO Quality of Life–Brief |

NOTES: AUDIT = Alcohol Use Disorders Identification Test; CI = confidence interval; DTI = diffusion tensor imaging; LOC = loss of consciousness; MRI = magnetic resonance imaging; OEF = Operation Enduring Freedom; OIF = Operation Iraqi Freedom; OR = odds ratio;

| Results | Adjustments | Comments or Limitations |
|---|---|---|
| PTSD severity associated with higher 1st percentile values of mean diffusivity on DTI (regression coefficient r = 4.2, p = 0.039), abnormal MRI (r = 13.3, p = 0.046), and severity of exposure to combat events (r = 5.4, p = 0.007). PTSD severity not associated with self-report of blast exposure. Blast exposure associated with lower 1st percentile values of fractional anisotropy on DTI (OR = 0.38 per SD; 95% CI, 0.15–0.92), normal MRI (OR = 0.00, 95% likelihood ratio test CI, 0.00–0.09), and severity of exposure to traumatic events (OR = 3.64 per SD; 95% CI, 1.40–9.43). Mild TBI not significantly associated with PTSD severity. | PTSD severity, mild TBI likelihood, severity of exposure to traumatic events, time since last tour of duty, prior head injury, age, sex | |
| Time 1: 9.2% mild TBI, 7.6% PTSD, 9.3% depression; time 2: 22% mild TBI, higher rates of PTSD and depression than time 1 (p < 0.001). Of those reporting a history of mild TBI at time 1, 30.2% had probable PTSD at time 2. Service members with a history of mild TBI were more likely than those without such symptoms to report postdeployment postconcussive symptoms and poorer psychosocial outcomes. After adjustment for PTSD symptoms, mild TBI was not associated with postdeployment postconcussive symptoms, depression, problematic drinking, nonspecific somatic complaints, social adjustment, or quality of life. | PTSD | No examination of moderate or severe TBI |

PTSD = posttraumatic stress disorder; SD = standard deviation; TBI = traumatic brain injury; WHO = World Health Organization.

outcomes more strongly than did mild TBI history. The results suggest that mild TBI alone does not result in long-term health outcomes as measured in this study.

The study is limited, however, in its usefulness in determining the long-term health effects of blast exposure because there was no direct comparison of those who had a blast-related injury with those who had a non-blast injury or no injury at all. Although many of those who reported symptoms of mild TBI, PTSD, or comorbid mild TBI and PTSD had a blast injury (mild TBI, 70%; PTSD, 35.9%; comorbid mild TBI and PTSD, 80%), it cannot be determined from the data analysis in the study whether a blast injury uniquely contributed to these health outcomes. Moreover, all outcome measures were based on self-reports and could have been affected by the service members' recall, amount of current distress, secondary gain, and so on. Because the survey participants were self-selected from a single brigade combat team and the survey had a low response rate of those who agreed to be contacted for participation in time 2 followup (50.4%), the findings may not be generalizable to all deployed military personnel. Finally, perhaps the most important limitation is that the time 1 assessment was conducted at the end of a 16-month deployment. The study would have been strengthened substantially if the time 1 assessment had been conducted before deployment so that the specific effects of deployment-related blast could be assessed (for example, concussion and mild TBI, PTSD, post-concussive symptoms, problem drinking, and depression).

Bazarian et al. (2013) conducted a nested cohort study to understand the relation of PTSD severity to mild TBI, blast exposure, and brain white matter structure. The participants were 52 Iraq and Afghanistan war veterans who served in combat areas during 2001–2008 and were studied about 4 years after their last tour of duty. Data on outcome measures were obtained from interview questions concerning blast exposure and TBI symptoms, the PTSD Checklist–Military, the Combat Experiences Scale, anatomic magnetic resonance imaging (MRI), and diffusion tensor imaging (DTI). The results of multivariate analyses demonstrated that PTSD severity was associated with higher 1st percentile values of mean diffusivity on DTI (regression coefficient $r = 4.2$, $p = 0 .039$), abnormal MRI ($r = 13.3$, $p = 0.046$), and severity of exposure to combat events ($r = 5.4$, $p = 0.007$). However, PTSD severity was not associated with self-reported blast exposure. Blast exposure was associated with lower 1st percentile values of fractional anisotropy on DTI (which is an abnormal DTI associated with PTSD severity) (odds ratio [OR] = 0.38 per standard deviation [SD]; 95% confidence interval [CI], 0.15–0.92), normal MRI (only five people had abnormalities on MRI, and 47 had normal results) (OR = 0.00, 95% likelihood ratio test CI, 0.00–0.09), and severity of exposure to traumatic events

(OR = 3.64 per SD; 95% CI, 1.40–9.43). Mild TBI was not significantly associated with PTSD severity.

The findings of the study showed that PTSD severity is related to the severity of combat stress and observed structural brain changes on MRI and DTI but not related to a clinical diagnosis of mild TBI. The observed relation between blast exposure and abnormal DTI suggests that subclinical TBI may play a role in the genesis of PTSD in a combat environment. The study demonstrates that asking questions about TBI symptoms may not be a good way to determine whether a person has suffered brain damage. The study was limited by its small sample and its use of self-reports of exposure.

## Supportive Studies

Four secondary studies provide some additional information on possible long-term psychological and psychiatric outcomes of blast exposure; however, each has limitations related to study design and the quantity and quality of information reported.

In a longitudinal cross-sectional and cohort study, Rona et al. (2012) conducted a questionnaire to assess the prevalence of mild TBI in UK military personnel deployed to Iraq and Afghanistan. They looked at risk factors associated with mild TBI and the association between mild TBI and postconcussive symptoms and other psychologic health outcomes. During 2007–2009, 4,620 personnel who had deployed to Iraq and Afghanistan completed the questionnaire in phase 2; 2,333 of them had been studied in 2005 (phase 1 predeployment health outcomes were observed in 2005 when the study was first established). Outcome measures included the reported incidence of mild TBI during deployment on the basis of a modified version of the Brief Traumatic Brain Injury Screen questionnaire and self-reported postconcussive symptoms that occurred in the month before the questionnaire was completed. Comorbid mental health conditions also were assessed with the PTSD checklist, General Health Questionaire–12, and AUDIT. Results showed that the overall prevalence of mild TBI was 4.4% and the prevalence in those who had a combat role, 9.5%. Having mild TBI was associated with current symptoms: PTSD (adjusted OR [AOR] = 5.2; 95% CI, 2.3–11.4), alcohol misuse (AOR = 2.3; 95% CI, 1.4–3.7), and multiple physical symptoms (AOR = 2.6; 95% CI, 1.3–5.2). Of those who had mild TBI with loss of consciousness, 46.8% reported that the mechanism of injury was blast. Of those who had mild TBI and altered mental status, 37.7% reported that the mechanism of injury was blast. No other comparison or analysis was done in this study to determine specific outcomes in blast- versus non-blast-injured people.

The study has limitations for the committee's determination of long-term psychologic outcomes of blast because of the data that were collected and the comparisons reported. For instance, the study did not report the average time between injury and reported health outcomes, so it is impossible to determine whether the observed outcomes were long-term consequences of injury or acute reactions. Another important limitation is that two samples were added in the phase 2 assessment because the authors were concerned that the followup sample would be too small. A separate longitudinal cohort analysis of the same samples before and after deployment would have strengthened the study.

Hoge et al. (2008) surveyed US Army infantry service members 3–4 months after their return from a year-long deployment to Iraq to compare service members who reported mild TBI with those who reported other injuries. Mild TBI was defined as a self-reported injury with loss of consciousness (LOC) or altered mental status (for example, being dazed or confused). Of 4,618 service members in two brigades who were asked to participate, 2,714 (59%) completed the questionnaire; 2,525 were then included in the study (others were screened out because of missing data or reports of head injury with no LOC or altered mental status). Findings showed that 79.0% of service members who suffered an injury with LOC were injured by blast exposure, 72.7% of those who had an injury with altered mental status were injured by blast, and only 23.2% of other reported injuries were due to blast. Service members who had mild TBI with LOC were significantly more likely to report poor general health, missed workdays, a high number of medical visits, and a high number of somatic and postconcussive symptoms than service members who had other injuries, such as moderate or severe TBI. However, after adjustment for PTSD and depression, mild TBI was no longer significantly associated with those physical health outcomes or symptoms, except for headache and heart pounding. Mild TBI was significantly associated with psychiatric symptoms such as those occurring with PTSD (more than 40% of service members who had injuries associated with LOC met criteria for PTSD). The study suggests that most of the postconcussive symptoms attributed to having previously experienced a blast-related mild TBI might actually be related to posttraumatic stress symptoms. Thus, the development of PTSD symptoms may be a long-term outcome of blast-induced mild TBI. However, analysis was not done to determine whether the blast mechanism of injury contributed uniquely to psychiatric symptoms as opposed to other mechanisms of injury. Although the study conducted surveys 3–4 months after deployment, it is impossible to know when the injuries took place and whether the reported symptoms were short-term or long-term symptoms.

As is also discussed in the section "Auditory and Vestibular Outcomes," Vanderploeg et al. (2012) conducted a cross-sectional cohort study that was based on data collected in anonymous online surveys to determine whether there was an association between military experience and immediate and long-term physical and psychologic health outcomes. The study also aimed to examine the effects of multiple deployment-related TBIs on health outcomes. The study included 3,098 members of the Florida National Guard (1,443 who had deployed and 1,655 who had not deployed). About 10,400 letters were mailed to solicit participation in the survey; 4,005 people completed the survey, and those who had been deployed completed it an average of 31.8 months (SD = 24.4 months, range = 0–95 months) after their deployment. ORs were calculated to assess the association between current health status and deployment-related factors, such as physical injuries, exposure to potentially traumatic deployment experiences, combat, blast exposure, and mild TBI. Demographics and predeployment experiences were controlled for as potential cofounders. The survey included a large number of questions to measure many predictors of health outcomes, such as blast exposure; of the 3,098 people in the study sample, 743 (24%) reported being exposed to blast. Results showed that deployment-related mild TBI was associated with depression, anxiety, PTSD, and postconcussive symptoms collectively and individually. There were also statistically significant increases in the frequency of depression, anxiety, PTSD, and a postconcussive symptom complex when people who had single incidents of TBI were compared with those who had multiple TBIs. A predeployment TBI did not appear to increase the likelihood of another TBI from a blast exposure. The experience of seeing others wounded or killed or experiencing the death of a fellow soldier or leader was associated with indigestion and headaches but not with depression, anxiety, or PTSD. The major limitations of this study are its cross-sectional design and its reliance on self-reported measures for all outcomes. In addition, the survey had a low response rate (41.3%), so the results shown here may not be generalizable to all deployed and nondeployed service members.

Finally, Bryant et al. (2009) conducted a longitudinal cohort study to examine the incidence of PTSD in a civilian population after nonmilitary traumatic injury in those who had mild TBI and those who had no TBI. Study participants were 1,167 survivors of traumatic injury (459 who had mild TBI and 708 who had no TBI) who were admitted to four level 1 trauma centers in Australia from April 2004 to February 2006. The subjects were assessed for PTSD symptoms and posttraumatic amnesia during hospitalization and then assessed for PTSD 3 months later. At the followup assessment, 90 (9.4%) of the 920 who were still participating met criteria for PTSD (mild TBI, 50, 11.8%; no TBI, 40, 7.5%). After controlling for injury severity, it was concluded that mild TBI patients were more likely to develop PTSD than no-TBI patients (AOR = 1.86; 95% CI, 1.78–2.94). Although the study is limited in its usefulness by its report outcomes only out to 3 months and not looking at blast injuries specifically, it adds to the evidence of a relationship between mild TBI and PTSD symptoms.

*Interventions to Mitigate the Long-Term Consequences of Blast*

A complete review of the treatment-outcome literature on combat-related PTSD is beyond the scope of the present report. However, a brief summary of the literature is helpful in determining the potential long-term consequences of PTSD. Historically, combat-related PTSD has been considered by many to be a chronic, lifelong condition that is difficult to treat. Indeed, combat-related PTSD in Vietnam veterans has been found to be a chronic disorder that fails to remit in almost 80% of cases evaluated decades after initial trauma exposure (Schnurr et al., 2003). Conversely, a recent long-term followup study of civilians treated with cognitive behavior therapy (cognitive processing therapy and prolonged exposure) indicated that about 80% of participants were treated to the point of remission and remained in remission for 5–10 years after participating in the study (Resick et al., 2012). Similar data on combat-related PTSD do not exist.

*Additional Psychologic and Psychiatric Consequences of Blast*

Scientific data on the relationship between exposure to blast and such mental disorders as major depressive disorder and substance-abuse disorders are fewer than data on the relationship between exposure to blast and PTSD. Depression and alcohol abuse are two of the most common mental-health comorbidities of PTSD. However, the relationship of depression to substance abuse separate from PTSD is not clear. The relationship of alcohol misuse to PTSD and depression symptoms was evaluated in a sample of 812 male US veterans of the Iraq war who had documented combat injuries (Heltemes et al., 2013). The results (after adjustment for age, rank, combat exposure, and mental health diagnosis before injury) indicated that veterans who had PTSD symptoms had significantly higher odds of reporting alcohol misuse than those who reported no PTSD symptoms (AOR = 4.05; 95% CI, 2.74–6.00). Veterans who had depression symptoms were also significantly more likely to have reported alcohol misuse than those who reported no depression symptoms (AOR = 4.22; 95% CI, 2.78–6.40).

## Conclusions

Relationships between multiple deployment-related factors and numerous overlapping and co-occurring adverse physical and psychologic health outcomes are complex. Acute psychologic and psychiatric outcomes of exposure to blast can include anxiety, depression, addiction, and worsening of existing psychiatric disorders. Two studies, considered primary by the committee, reported an association between exposure to blast and PTSD; this finding has been corroborated by several supportive studies.

The associations between exposure to blast and other chronic mental health outcomes, such as depression and substance-use disorders, are less well understood.

> The committee concludes, on the basis of its evaluation, that there is sufficient evidence of an association between exposure to blast and posttraumatic stress disorder. The association may be related to direct experience of blast or to indirect exposure, such as witnessing the aftermath of a blast or being part of a community affected by a blast.

> The committee concludes, on the basis of its evaluation, that there is sufficient evidence of a substantial overlap in the symptoms of mild traumatic brain injury (TBI) and posttraumatic stress disorder (PTSD) after exposure to blast. Furthermore, the committee concludes, on the basis of its evaluation, that there is limited/suggestive evidence that most of the shared symptoms are accounted for by PTSD and are not a direct result of TBI alone.

> The committee concludes, on the basis of its evaluation, that there is inadequate/insufficient evidence to assess the direct contribution of blast to depression, substance-use disorders, and chronic pain; however, the association of posttraumatic stress disorder with these disorders is well established.

## NERVOUS SYSTEM OUTCOMES

TBI is the dominant blast injury that affects the nervous system. The Department of Veterans Affairs (VA) and the Department of Defense (DOD) define TBI as "traumatically induced structural injury and/or a physiological disruption of brain function as a result of an external force," with at least one of the following manifestations: decreased level of consciousness, loss of memory immediately before or after the injury, alteration in mental state, neurological deficits, or intracranial lesions (Shively and Perl, 2012). TBI severity is generally classified into three tiers: mild, moderate, and severe. The VA and DOD shared guidelines for distinguishing TBI severity are based on the following criteria: structural imaging, LOC, alteration of consciousness (AOC), posttraumatic amnesia (PTA), and the Glasgow Coma Scale (GCS) (VA and DOD, 2009). The GCS is a severity score itself; it is aggregated from performance ratings of eye opening, motor response, and verbal response and has been the gold standard of neurologic assessment of trauma patients since its development by Teasdale and Jennett in 1974 (see Table 4-2) (IOM, 2009; Teasdale and Jennett, 1974). VA and DOD define mild TBI as presenting with one or more of the following: nor-

**TABLE 4-2** Severity Scoring of the Glasgow Coma Scale

| Response | Degree of Response | Score |
|---|---|---|
| Eye opening | Spontaneous—open with blinking at baseline | 4 |
| | To verbal stimuli, command, speech | 3 |
| | To pain only (not applied to face) | 2 |
| | No response | 1 |
| Best verbal response | Oriented | 5 |
| | Confused conversation, but able to answer questions | 4 |
| | Inappropriate words | 3 |
| | Incomprehensible speech | 2 |
| | No response | 1 |
| Best motor response | Obeys commands for movement | 6 |
| | Purposeful movement to painful stimulus | 5 |
| | Withdraws in response to pain | 4 |
| | Flexion response to pain (decorticate posturing) | 3 |
| | Extension response to pain (decerebrate posturing) | 2 |
| | No response | 1 |

SOURCE: Adapted from Teasdale and Jennett (1976) with permission from Springer Science and Business Media.

mal structural imaging, LOC duration of 0–30 minutes, AOC duration of a moment to 24 hours, PTA duration less than 24 hours, and a GCS score of 13–15. Moderate TBI is defined by one or more of the following: normal or abnormal structural imaging, LOC duration of 30 minutes–24 hours, AOC duration greater than 24 hours, PTA duration of 24 hours–1 week, and a GCS score of 9–12. Severe TBI is defined by one or more of the following: normal or abnormal structural imaging, LOC and AOC lasting more than 24 hours, PTA lasting more than 1 week, and a GCS score less than 9 (VA and DOD, 2009). That schema incorporates the most widely adopted case definition of mild TBI provided by the American Congress of Rehabilitative Medicine (ACRM, 1993) and the consensus among the scientific community of the case definitions of moderate and severe TBI (Sayer, 2012).

From January 1, 2000, to August 20, 2012, a total of 253,330 US service members—of the 2.2 million deployed—had a diagnosis of TBI while serving in the Iraq and Afghanistan wars (Fischer, 2013). Most (77%) of the cases were mild. Exposure to blast can cause TBI through primary, secondary, tertiary, and quaternary mechanisms. Evidence from clinical experience and experimental neuroimaging suggests that TBI caused by blast waves (blast TBI) is distinct from TBI caused by closed head injuries due to blunt trauma and from penetrating TBI (Magnuson et al., 2012).

Studies of TBI have been conducted in nearly all the major conflicts of the 20th century, including World Wars I and II, the Korean War, and the Vietnam War; many of the studies evaluated seizure as the outcome of interest. For example, during the Vietnam War, 12–14% of all combat casualties had a TBI (Okie, 2005). However, the populations in those studies had penetrating and severe closed head injuries and the mechanisms of injury are not typically reported. A detailed summary of studies of TBI (not specifically related to exposure to blast) in veteran populations can be found in *Gulf War and Health, Volume 7: Long-Term Consequences of Traumatic Brain Injury* (IOM, 2009).

## Acute Effects

Mild blast TBI can cause acute headache, anxiety, vertigo, sleep disturbance, mood alteration, and a cognitive deficit that includes confusion, brief LOC, amnesia, short-term memory loss, and difficulty in concentrating (Brenner et al., 2012; Magnuson et al., 2012). Those effects may resolve in a matter of a few days; one study showed that in a civilian population exposed to mild closed-head-injury TBI, symptoms had resolved in most patients at a 1-year followup (Alexander, 1995). In rare circumstances, however, symptoms can fluctuate in severity or be unapparent immediately after the injury, only to be triggered by life stressors months later (Hicks et al., 2010). Mild blast TBI is clinically indistinguishable from other types of mild TBI at this level of severity, and the outcomes mentioned here may occur from secondary, tertiary, and quaternary effects of the blast as well. A particular danger with mild TBI is that service members may ignore or endure the milder symptoms and then expose themselves to a second blast, putting themselves at risk of second-impact syndrome. Outcomes can be more severe if someone already suffering from mild TBI is subjected to a second concussion. Second-impact syndrome can present with prolonged LOC, malignant cerebral edema, and coma. Although it is extremely rare, the risk of second-impact syndrome may be greater in patients who are exposed to blast than in those who have other types of trauma (Armonda et al., 2006). It is associated with up to 50% mortality (Magnuson et al., 2012).

Moderate to severe blast TBI can cause hemorrhage, skull fracture, cerebral edema, and parenchymal contusions which are all easily detectable with neuroimaging. Patients present with acute effects ranging from confusion and lethargy to coma and even death (Magnuson et al., 2012). Differences in diffuse axonal injury between blast TBI and closed head-injury TBI can be observed at this level of severity with advanced neuroimaging techniques (Davenport et al., 2012). Brains exposed to blast TBI can develop malignant cerebral edema faster (in less than 1 hour) than those exposed to closed-head-injury TBI (in several hours to 1 day) (Magnuson et al., 2012). Cerebral vasospasm, which may lead to secondary cerebral infarction days after the injury, may be prolonged, with a duration after blast TBI twice that after closed-head-injury TBI (Oertel et al., 2005).

Two less understood outcomes that can occur with TBI of any type or severity are seizures and posttraumatic epilepsy. The latter is defined as the occurrence of two or more seizures more than 7 days after a blast; it is more frequent after more severe episodes of TBI (Magnuson et al., 2012). Seizures can be manifested with only mild behavioral and cognitive alterations, so in some settings it may be difficult to detect without electroencephalographic monitoring (Magnuson et al., 2012).

Of particular difficulty in determining the neurologic effects of blast TBI is that these often develop in the polytrauma setting. Patients who have TBI from blast frequently also suffer damage to neurosensory organs, such as the ears and eyes, and to solid organs (such as the heart and lungs); all these injuries can have direct and indirect influences on brain function. The Defense and Veterans Brain Injury Center found that 66% of TBI patients seen at Walter Reed Army Medical Center (WRAMC) over a 2-year period also suffered ocular trauma (Magnuson et al., 2012). Another study retrospectively evaluating 10,341 victims of blast TBI concluded that 68.5% had concomitant hearing impairment (Lew et al., 2011). It can be difficult to ascertain which neurologic symptoms are directly related to blast TBI itself and which are related to other kinds of injury from the blast that affects the nervous system secondarily.

Neurologic effects of blast to the inner ear may take the form of centrally or peripherally mediated disequilibrium, vertigo, posttraumatic Ménière disease, and sensorineural hearing loss (Magnuson et al., 2012; Scherer et al., 2007). Penetrating or severe nonpenetrating forces on the eye can cause optic nerve damage that results in impairment or loss of vision (Morley et al., 2010). Damage to the cardiovascular system caused by blast injury can compromise blood supply to the brain and cause generalized cerebral dysfunction, such as altered affect, confusion, disorientation, or focal neurologic signs from stroke, traumatic cerebral vasospasm, arterial air emboli, or arterial dissection (Magnuson et al., 2012; Phillips, 1986). Musculoskeletal injury and damage to the spinal cord and vertebrae caused by blast can result in paralysis (Eardley et al., 2012). Bone fractures and other crush injuries or compartment syndromes may result in peripheral nerve palsies or muscle damage at the site of injury (Scott et al., 1986).

## Long-Term Effects

Some acute injuries to the central nervous system (CNS) will never resolve. Spinal cord injuries that result in paralysis, incontinence, or loss of ability to breathe spontaneously often will be permanent. Cerebral contusions and other structural brain injuries may lead to permanent neurologic dysfunction, including posttraumatic epilepsy; in one study, 19% of patients who suffered moderate to severe TBI had epilepsy at a 10-year followup (Andelic et al., 2009).

The committee that prepared *Gulf War and Health, Volume 7: Long-Term Consequences of Traumatic Brain Injury* (IOM, 2009) concluded that there was sufficient evidence of a causal relationship between

- Penetrating TBI and unprovoked seizures.
- Penetrating TBI and premature death.
- Severe or moderate TBI and unprovoked seizures.

It concluded further that there was sufficient evidence of an association between

- Penetrating TBI and a decline in cognitive function.
- Penetrating TBI and long-term unemployment.
- Severe TBI and cognitive deficits.
- Severe or moderate TBI and dementia of the Alzheimer type.[1]
- Severe or moderate TBI and parkinsonism.
- Severe or moderate TBI and endocrine dysfunction (hypopituitarism and growth hormone deficiency).
- Severe or moderate TBI and adverse social-function outcomes.
- Severe or moderate TBI and premature death.
- All forms of TBI and depression, aggressive behaviors, and post-concussive symptoms.[2]

In the studies examined in the 2009 Institute of Medicine (IOM) report and other studies of TBI that have followed, both blast and non-blast mechanisms of TBI have been combined in analyses. In instances where there would be no likely difference in consequences between blast and non-blast TBI, the present committee used data from the studies to help to determine the relationship between blast exposure and long-term neurologic effects. However, given the animal and other data that suggest potentially unique, and in some cases more severe, injuries to the nervous system caused by blast exposure compared with TBI caused by other mechanisms (see Chapter 3), the committee also sought to identify studies that focused on blast-related TBI.

---

[1] Studies published after the release of the 2009 report show that the association between severe or moderate TBI and dementia is likely due to a mixture of pathologies rather than solely Alzheimer Disease.

[2] The association between TBI and aggressive behaviors has been shown for the severe and moderate forms of TBI.

To evaluate the long-term neurologic effects of blast exposure, the committee reviewed about 50 published peer-reviewed studies. It did not find any studies that met the inclusion guidelines for primary studies. This section details the identified supportive studies of long-term neurologic health outcomes of blast exposure.

*Chronic Traumatic Encephalopathy*

One recently recognized long-term effect of repeated TBI is chronic traumatic encephalopathy (CTE), a slowly progressive neurodegenerative disorder that usually does not present until 8–10 years after the exposure and is characterized pathologically by progressive accumulation of abnormal (hyperphosphorylated) deposits of tau protein in neurons and associated atrophy of brain tissue (McKee et al., 2012). Initial symptoms include irritability, impulsivity, aggression, depression, sleep disruption, memory loss, and heightened suicidality, all of which can clinically resemble common forms of dementia. CTE has been observed in professional athletes, especially American football players. However, little is known about the prevalence of CTE in the blast-injured population or even about whether it can occur after single blast TBI episodes. Goldstein et al. (2012) examined brains from three military personnel who were known to be exposed to blast and found CTE-linked neuropathologic characteristics: perivascular foci of tau-immunoreactive neurofibrillary tangles and glial tangles in the inferior frontal, dorsolateral frontal, parietal, and temporal cortices with a predilection for sulcal depths.

*Headache*

Headache is the most common disorder in most neurology clinics and among the three most common in general-medicine clinics. Migraine is the secondmost common type of headache; 15% of women and 6% of men in the general population experience migraine in a 1-year period (Stewart et al., 1994). Tension headache is four times as common as migraine. In the general population, 4% of adults have chronic daily headache (CDH), defined as headache on at least 15 days per month; this entity is not a single condition, and in the general population as much as 15% of cases of CDH may be attributable to some sort of head trauma (Couch et al., 2007). Headache is a common sequela of a diverse set of head-trauma mechanisms in clinical experience, so it is likely to result also from blast exposure.

The committee identified three secondary studies. In a retrospective cohort study of 91 service members from the same brigade who had chronic headache after a 1-year combat tour in Iraq, 41% had a history of head and neck trauma during their tour, and 67% of the traumas were due to blast (Theeler and Erickson, 2009). In one-third of the patients with head and neck trauma, a new headache started after the trauma; in an additional one-third, a preexisting headache worsened after the trauma. Migraine was the most common headache type identified. Limitations of the study include the small sample, the retrospective design, and selection bias (a clinic-based population was assessed).

In a cross-sectional study of service members undergoing postdeployment health evaluation, those with a self-identified history of concussion received a specific headache questionnaire (Theeler et al., 2010). Some 20% of the 5,270 service members deployed to Iraq or Afghanistan who were studied met criteria for deployment-related concussion, and 37% experienced posttraumatic headache. Migraine was the most common phenotype seen. The study did not address the mechanism of concussion, although in many cases it probably was blast. The contribution of PTSD and psychiatric disorders was not detailed in the study. There were several limitations related to the questionnaire-based, cross-sectional design of the study, including recall error and possible misclassification of headache type.

In a cross-sectional study of 978 service members deployed to Iraq or Afghanistan who screened positive for postdeployment concussion headache, 196 were found to have CDH with a median of 27 headache days per month (Theeler et al., 2012). In 55% of the CDH patients, the headaches began within 1 week of concussion, compared with 33% of those who reported episodic headache. Two-thirds of those who had CDH met criteria for migraine. No differences were found between the CDH and episodic-headache groups in the number of blast exposures, concussions, or concussions with LOC. The CHD patients had significantly higher scores than the episodic-headache group on a PTSD checklist; this emphasizes the link between PTSD and CDH after blast exposure. The cross-sectional design of the study constitutes a limitation because reports of CDH and of blast exposure are retrospectively self-reported, and there may be recall error. In addition, it was not known whether any of the subjects experienced CDH before blast exposure.

Another study, considered tertiary by the committee, found that among 126 Iraq and Afghanistan war veterans who experienced exposure to blast and sustained a mild TBI, nearly two-thirds (80) had frequent severe headaches, usually with migrainous features, accompanied by PTSD and impaired sleep with nightmares (Ruff et al., 2008).

*Endocrine Changes*

Blast injury may affect the pituitary gland and thus disrupt hormonal function. Two secondary studies were identified to support that idea. Wilkinson et al. (2012) studied 26 Iraq and Afghanistan war veterans who were exposed to blast at least 1 year before testing and compared them with 59 veterans who do not have blast exposure. Eleven of the blast group (and none of the non-blast group) had abnormal hormone concentrations in one or more pituitary axes. Half of those patients had abnormalities of anterior pituitary function, and half had posterior pituitary abnormalities. Five patients were growth hormone deficient, and three suffered from hypogonadism. Baxter et al. (2013) studied endocrine function in 19 UK service members who served in the Afghanistan war and had moderate to severe blast TBI. The service members underwent MRI, including DTI, and cognitive assessment. Control subjects were civilians who had moderate to severe nonblast TBI. Anterior pituitary dysfunction was found in 6 (32%) of the 19 service members who had blast TBI and 1 of the 39 controls (p = 0.004). The service members who had pituitary dysfunction had greater traumatic axonal injury in the cerebellum and corpus callosum, more skull and facial fractures, and worse cognitive function than the service members who did not have pituitary dysfunction.

## Postconcussive Symptoms

After TBI, patients often experience a variety of persistent postconcussive symptoms including headache (discussed on page 102), difficulty in concentrating, aggressiveness, and irritability. The committee identified three secondary studies that described postconcussive symptoms after exposure to blast.

In a study of 339 veterans of the Iraq and Afghanistan wars who had a history of mild TBI, posttraumatic stress symptoms were found to be significantly worse in the blast and mixed (blast plus non-blast) groups than in the group that had only non-blast mechanisms (Lippa et al., 2010). PTSD-like symptoms accounted for 47% of the variance in the postconcussive symptoms.

In a study of 91 Iraq and Afghanistan war veterans who had a history of being within 100 m of a blast, veterans who had TBI and LOC had significantly more postconcussive symptoms than those who did not have TBI or those who had TBI without LOC (Verfaellie et al., 2013). However, after adjustment for depressive and PTSD symptoms, the result was no longer significant. The mild TBI with LOC group had greater psychosocial limitations than the other groups, and this relationship persisted even after adjustment for depressive and PTSD symptoms. The relationship between postconcussive symptoms and Axis I psychiatric disorders has been well detailed in previous studies not specific to blast injury.

In a study of structured interviews that attempt to associate blast-related TBI with neuropsychologic outcomes, 18 veterans of the Iraq and Afghanistan wars who experienced mild TBI were compared with those who had only Axis I disorders (24 veterans), those who had mild TBI and Axis I disorders (34 veterans), and postdeployment controls; no difference was found between the mild-TBI group and the other groups (Nelson et al., 2012b). Limitations of the study include the lack of addressing the contribution of PTSD and the fact that some blast exposures reported in interviews with the veterans were minor and did not lead to concussions.

Seven additional studies were considered tertiary by the committee, but provided some further information about exposure to blast and post-concussive symptoms. Trudeau et al. (1998) reported that combat veterans who had a remote history of blast injury (27 veterans) have persistent electroencephalographic features that are consistent with TBI and attention problems. Kennedy et al. (2010) found that 130 US Iraq and Afghanistan war service members who had mild TBI but no other associated physical injuries had higher symptom ratings than those who had mild TBI and associated physical injuries (144 service members); one explanation for this result might be that patients who have physical injuries can focus on making progress toward healing and functional improvement whereas patients who have only mild TBI experience somatic neuropsychologic symptoms. Heltemes et al. (2012) found that 473 US service members who sustained blast-related mild TBI self-reported adverse changes in health 6 months after injury 5 times more often than did 656 service members who sustained other types of injuries. Scheibel et al. (2012) conducted a stimulus-response compatibility task by using functional magnetic resonance imaging (fMRI) on 15 US service personnel and veterans of the Iraq and Afghanistan wars who had blast-related mild TBI and compared them with 15 controls who did not have TBI and were not exposed to blast. The subjects who had experienced blast-related mild TBI demonstrated slower fMRI responses and increased symptoms of PTSD, depression, and somatic complaints. Another neuroimaging study used a magnetoencephalographic low-frequency source imaging method and demonstrated abnormalities in 96% of 23 blast-exposed mild TBI patients and 77% of 22 non-blast mild TBI patients (Huang et al., 2012). Walker et al. (2013) reported that 29 (33.3%) of 87 US service personnel and veterans who served in Iraq and Afghanistan reported at least one of three concrete alteration-of-consciousness items—gap in memory (17.2%), memory not continuous (13.8%), and being told by an observer that they had LOC (20.7%)—after experiencing acute effects of blast exposure within the preceeding 2 years; these results again suggest that mild TBI plays a role in the development of chronic neuropsychiatric symptoms after exposure to blast. Mendez et al. (2013) studied changes in personality in 12 US veterans who had blast-related mild TBI and 12 US veterans who experienced blunt-force mild TBI and found that, on the basis of select measures of personality, veterans who had blast-related mild TBI had more negative personality changes than those who had blunt-force mild TBI.

### Cognitive Changes

Several reported studies have many limitations and were considered tertiary by the committee but provide some information about cognitive effects related to blast exposure. Cooper et al. (2012) conducted a retrospective review to assess neurocognitive function in 32 Iraq and Afghanistan–war service members who had blast-related mild TBI and 28 who had nonblast-related mild TBI about 6 months after injury and did not find significant differences between the groups in any neurocognitive domain. Coldren et al. (2012) administered the automated neuropsychiatric assessment metric within 10 days of injury to 47 concussed and 108 non-concussed service members who served in Iraq and Afghanistan; concussed service members were more likely to have been exposed to a blast. The neurocognitive changes found with the metric were not reassessed later. Mac Donald et al. (2011) used DTI and found cerebellar abnormalities consistent with traumatic axonal injury in 18 (29%) of 63 US service members who had TBI and self-reported blast exposure; by chance alone, only two of 63 healthy subjects would be expected to have such abnormalities. Matthews et al. (2011) performed a stop-task-based fMRI on 27 US Iraq and Afghanistan–war service members and found that subjects who had a history of LOC had altered ventromedial prefrontal cortex activity more than subjects who had a history only of alteration of consciousness; this finding correlated with the severity of somatic symptoms experienced and suggested a neural correlate of impaired self-awareness after LOC. Finally, Sponheim et al. (2011) used electroencephalography phase synchronization and DTI to assess nine service members who were deployed to Iraq and Afghanistan and suffered blast-related mild TBI; they did not report cognitive deficits but observed more frequent electroencephalographic abnormalities in frontal and lateral cerebral regions and problems with structural integrity of frontal white-matter tracts than in controls, persisting after controlling for PTSD, depression, and medications.

Advanced neuroimaging (for example, DTI and fMRI) has led to several insights regarding the cognitive effects of TBI in veterans. DTI studies have revealed evidence of disruptions of CNS tracts suggestive of TBI in bodily injured service members even in the absence of reported history of TBI (Xydakis et al., 2012). That suggests that the true incidence of anatomically significant TBI may not be captured by using routine clinical and imaging criteria, especially in critically injured service members. The history typical of concussion ("seeing stars" and LOC) may not be present with blast TBI, so additional neuroimaging studies may be required for this diagnosis. Changes in DTI have been found in some studies of blast-associated TBI. For example, Mac Donald et al. (2011) found changes consistent with multifocal traumatic axonal injury in a group of seriously injured service members who were exposed to blast events and who had normal computed tomography scans; evolution of the changes 6–12 months later revealed persistence and some dynamic changes that were compatible with evolution of the acute lesions. DTI changes were also found with mild TBI in studies by Davenport et al. (2012), Jorge et al. (2012), and Matthews et al. (2012) but not by Levin et al. (2010). Technical differences may account for those discrepancies, and recent technical advances focusing on identifying spatially heterogeneous areas of decreased functional anisotropy ("potholes") suggest that this method may be more sensitive in determining TBI severity and impaired executive functioning. The axonal injury that is persistent in chronic cases may create a potential surrogate identifier for a TBI event, which is especially important because the usual criteria used to recognize mild TBI may not be present or may be obscured by other bodily injuries.

Using DTI, Davenport et al. (2012) studied 25 Iraq and Afghanistan war veterans who had blast-related TBI and 33 veterans who did not have blast exposure and found global disruption of white-matter tracts in the blast-exposed veterans. No differences were found in more concentrated white-matter regions. A history of prior civilian mild TBI did not affect the results. The injury appeared to be dose dependent inasmuch as greater numbers of blast exposures were associated with a larger number of low voxels when fractional anisotropy was used. Another study of 12 Iraq war veterans who had persistent postconcussive symptoms and healthy community volunteers showed decreased metabolism in the veterans on the basis of fluorodeoxyglucose positron emission tomography in the cerebellum, pons, and medial temporal lobe; those who had mild TBI also had subtle impairments in verbal fluency, cognitive processing speed, attention, and working memory on neuropsychologic testing (Peskind et al., 2011). A limitation is that the volunteer controls were an average of 20 years older than the veterans, although the deficits identified on imaging and neuropsychologic testing in the younger veterans would be more likely to increase with age, so this potential bias is less likely to explain the results.

## Spinal Injuries

The committee identified two secondary studies of spinal injuries associated with exposure to blast. Comstock et al. (2011) found that improvised explosive devices (IEDs) are more likely to cause spinal injuries than are other mechanisms, such as blunt trauma. Through the Joint Theatre Trauma Registry (JTTR) 372 Canadian Forces personnel who served in Afghanistan and were injured during the period February 7, 2006–October

14, 2009, were identified and included in the study. Of the 372, 212 (57%) were injured by IEDs, and 29 (8%) had spinal fractures. Members injured by IEDs were significantly more likely to have spinal injuries than those injured by non-blast mechanisms (10.4% vs 2.3%). A major limitation of the study is that the researchers were unable to conduct a detailed chart review of most of the patients' medical records and were unable to ascertain details of the injuries, such as type of fracture, neurologic findings, and functional outcome.

Blair et al. (2012) used the JTTR to identify US military personnel of the Iraq and Afghanistan wars from October 2001 through December 2009 who sustained back, spinal column, and spinal cord injuries. Of 10,979 combat casualties, 598 (5.45%) sustained 2,101 injuries to the spinal column or spinal cord; 92% of these injuries were fractures. Of the 598 patients, 336 (56%) were injured by exposure to blast. Of the 104 patients who had spinal cord injuries, 38 (36.5%) were injured by exposure to blast. Limitations of the study include reliance on JTTR data, which can be incomplete, especially during the early years of the wars, and the fact that medical records of service members killed in action are not included in the JTTR.

Three additional studies, considered tertiary by the committee, provided further evidence about spinal injuries due to blast exposure. Ragel et al. (2009) conducted a retrospective analysis of North Atlantic Treaty Organization service members who sustained spine fractures when riding in vehicles attacked by IEDs. Twelve patients who had 16 thoracolumbar fractures were identified, and 6 of the fractures were flexion–distraction thoracolumbar fractures; most spine-fracture series report the prevalence of flexion–distraction thoracolumbar fractures as 1.0–2.5%, so these injuries may be characteristic of IED explosions. Bell et al. (2009) conducted a retrospective review of 513 inpatient admissions in the Iraq war from April 2003 to April 2008 that were evaluated at the National Naval Medical Center and WRAMC. Of the 513, 56% were injured by exposure to blast, and 408 had either a closed or a penetrating head injury, including 40 who also had a spinal column injury, but the number of patients who had spinal column injuries and were exposed to blast is not reported. Using the Armed Forces Medical Examiner System, Schoenfeld et al. (2013) identified 5,424 deceased military personnel who had been deployed to Iraq and Afghanistan from 2003 to 2011 and sustained a spinal injury in conjunction with wounds that resulted in death; 67% of all fatalities with spinal injury were attributed to exposure to blast.

## Conclusions

Acute short-term effects of TBI were well described in *Gulf War and Health, Volume 7: Long-Term Consequences of Traumatic Brain Injury* (IOM, 2009). Permanent neurologic disability—including cognitive dysfunction, unprovoked seizures, and headache—is causally related to moderate or severe TBI. Those clinical syndromes result from the known pathologic conditions associated with nonpenetrating impact injuries, including fractures, hemorrhages, contusions, and brain swelling. The present committee was not able to identify primary studies that focused exclusively on acute blast-related TBI. However, inasmuch as many of the studies cited in *Volume 7* included both blast and non-blast TBI, it is likely that the injuries are at least as severe in blast TBI, although further research is required to determine whether there are additional unique patterns of injury. Moreover, secondary and tertiary blast effects due to fragments of debris and acceleration and deceleration injuries, respectively, result from primary blast effects, and it is expected that the secondary and tertiary injuries will resemble missile and concussive injuries seen in other settings. Although the clinical and pathologic syndromes of blast-induced TBI and other forms of TBI probably overlap extensively, there may be some differences that could potentially produce distinctive presentations and require different therapeutic strategies. For example, typical symptoms of concussion, such as seeing stars and experiencing a transient LOC, may be absent. The limited evidence indicates that early malignant brain swelling, sometimes referred to as second-impact syndrome, may be more common in connection with blast than with other injuries (Armonda et al., 2006). In addition, numerous studies have suggested that blast TBI may confer distinctive neuroimaging patterns as measured by DTI (tractography). In blast injury, a diffuse bihemispheric pattern of disruption may occur, unlike the more focal, often frontal and occipital (coup–contracoup) pattern classically observed in acceleration–deceleration concussive injury. That pattern could potentially result in a higher frequency of global cerebral complaints involving cognitive, visual, auditory, and other sensory modalities in those exposed to blast; however, the evidence confirming these distinctive mechanisms is preliminary and insufficient to permit any firm conclusions to be drawn.

**The committee concludes, on the basis of its evaluation, that there is sufficient evidence of an association between severe or moderate blast-related traumatic brain injury and endocrine dysfunction (hypopituitarism and growth hormone deficiency).**

The committee concludes, on the basis of its evaluation, that there is sufficient evidence of an association between mild blast traumatic brain injury and postconcussive symptoms and persistent headache.

The committee concludes, on the basis of its evaluation, that there is limited/suggestive evidence of an association between recurrent blast traumatic brain injury and chronic traumatic encephalopathy with progressive cognitive and behavioral decline.

The committee concludes, on the basis of its evaluation, that there is limited/suggestive evidence that diffuse brain injury with swelling may be more likely after blast than in relation to other mechanisms that lead to traumatic brain injury.

The committee concludes, on the basis of its evaluation, that in other brain-injury mechanisms (non-blast traumatic brain injury [TBI]), there is sufficient evidence of an association between severe or moderate TBI and permanent neurologic disability, including cognitive dysfunction, unprovoked seizures, and headache. These associations also are known outcomes in TBI studies that included blast and non-blast mechanisms considered together. It is plausible that severe or moderate blast TBI is similarly associated with permanent neurologic disability even though studies that specifically addressed blast TBI are lacking.

## AUDITORY AND VESTIBULAR OUTCOMES

The ear is typically one of the first organs to sustain damage from a blast event and is the organ most susceptible to primary blast injury (Jagade et al., 2008; Phillips and Richmond, 1991). Injury to the external ear is possible from secondary, tertiary, and quaternary blast exposure, but primary blast injury to the middle and inner ear is much more common and likely to affect auditory function. Traditionally, clinical attention has focused on tympanic membrane (TM) perforations, hearing loss, and tinnitus complaints as the primary manifestations of auditory dysfunction after blast exposure. However, those clinical outcomes do not adequately capture the array of auditory dysfunction that may be associated with acute trauma from blast. Normal auditory function requires an intact ear (especially middle and inner ear) but also relies on the complex signal transduction, transmission, and processing mechanisms that are involved in centrally translating and integrating sounds. Blast—through its effects on the microcirculation, apoptosis, shearing of neural networks, and other mechanisms—may have additional implications for the auditory system and the processing of auditory information, especially in complex environments.

Although loud noise from such exposures as gunfire may cause damage to the auditory system, the focus of this review is on blast injuries.

## Acute Effects

Perforation of the TM is the most common form of injury to the middle ear (Jagade et al., 2008). The TM is extremely sensitive to pressure (its primary function is to sense vibrations in sound waves), so it is highly susceptible to blast overpressure. Some cases of TM perforation close spontaneously over weeks to months after blast exposure. Much less common in the middle ear—especially after small to medium blasts—is disruption of the ossicular chain. Patients who have sustained damage to the middle ear from primary blast injury may present with earache and conductive hearing loss, which may be temporary and resolve with the healing of the TM (Jagade et al., 2008; Walsh et al., 1995). It is possible that cholesteatoma and infection can develop from a primary blast injury to the middle ear and potentially lead to erosion and destruction of important structures of the middle ear, temporal bone, and skull casing (Jagade et al., 2008).

Primary blast injuries to the inner ear involve the disruption of the vestibular apparatus and cochlea and can result in sensorineural hearing loss due to temporary or permanent damage to the hair cells of the cochlea, which are the delicate sensory structures responsible for amplification of sound and its transduction to the auditory nerve and central auditory nervous system (Finlay et al., 2012). The inner ear can be directly affected by the blast or indirectly affected by sequelae of injury to the middle ear.

## Long-Term Effects

Although the symptoms of blast ear injury often resolve spontaneously, they may also be chronic or permanent. Tinnitus and hearing loss are the two most prevalent medical disability claims in VA (2011).

To evaluate the long-term auditory and vestibular health effects of blast exposure, the committee reviewed about 80 published peer-reviewed studies. Seven met the committee's guidelines for primary studies (see Table 4-3). Of the seven, only two reported outcomes of blast during military deployment. The others were studies of civilian exposure to blast. This section details the identified primary and supportive studies of long-term auditory and vestibular outcomes due to blast exposure.

### Primary Studies

Several of the studies identified as primary by the committee involved health outcomes in survivors of the Oklahoma City bombing on April 19,

**TABLE 4-3** Auditory Outcomes—Primary Studies

| Reference | Study Design | Population | Health Outcomes or Outcome Measures |
|---|---|---|---|
| Cohen et al., 2002 | Cohort | 17 survivors of a suicide terrorist explosion on bus in Israel, followed for 6 months; 7 males and 10 females; median age 28 years; October 1994–April 1995 | Auditory, vestibular, otoneurologic evaluations |
| Riviere et al., 2008 | Cohort | 103 blast-exposed workers at a chemical plant in France, 91.3% men, 39.9 ± 8.5 years old vs 105 "less-exposed" workers (defined by distance ≥ 1,700 m from blast), 79.1% men, 39.8 ± 8.6 years old; required routine audiometric test since 1990 and before the explosion in September 2001 | Pure-tone air conduction audiometric test, conducted 1 month–3 years after blast vs before blast |
| Shariat et al., 1999 | Cohort assembled from registry created by Oklahoma State Department of Health | 494 survivors of 1995 Oklahoma City bombing, 92% of whom had sustained physical injuries and were treated in hospital or received outpatient care | Long-term physical and emotional outcomes assessed 1.5–3 years after blast via telephone interview |

| Results | Adjustments | Comments or Limitations |
|---|---|---|
| At 6 months, 73.3% aural fullness, 71.4% dizziness, 40.0% tinnitus, 22.3% otalgia, 44.4% perforated eardrums. Hearing loss: 44.1% SNHL, 8.8% CHL, 26.4% MHL, 20.5% normal. CDP abnormal 46.1%. ENG abnormal 0%. Of 7 cases with vestibular complaints, 4 had multisensory dysfunction on CDP, 1 had vestibular loss. | None | No control group. |
| Blast wave equivalent to 3.4-magnitude earthquake. Minimum peak acoustic levels estimated to be 160–194 dB (2–100 kPa) within 1,700 m. 19.5% of exposed workers reported functional symptoms of otalgia, vertigo, tinnitus, or other. Right ear (exposed vs "less exposed"): hearing loss at 2,000 Hz (p < 0.05), 4,000 Hz (p < 0.001), borderline at 6,000 Hz (p = 0.09). Left ear: hearing loss at 2,000 Hz (p < 0.01), 6,000 Hz (p < 0.05), 8,000 Hz (p < 0.05). | Age, sex, history of ear problems, past occupational noise exposure, period between two audiograms | Precise time of audio testing relative to time of explosion not specified; could have been 1–3 years. Specificity of symptoms not reported; only total percentage with *any* symptoms is reported; p values in Table 1 not the same as those in abstract. |
| Auditory problems were most common health outcome. 32% of cohort reported newly diagnosed auditory problems since bombing; 44% reported "ringing/ roaring in ears"; 40% reported "trouble hearing." Hospitalized survivors reported more hearing problems than those who had less severe injuries. 9% of uninjured or not treated patients reported newly diagnosed auditory problem; 48% of cohort used audiology services. | | Self-reported data; no control group. |

*continued*

**TABLE 4-3** Continued

| Reference | Study Design | Population | Health Outcomes or Outcome Measures |
|---|---|---|---|
| Van Campen et al., 1999a | Longitudinal cohort | 83 survivors of 1995 Oklahoma City bombing; mean age 43 years, 45% female and 55% male, evaluated 4 times over 1 year vs 10 healthy subjects, 50% female and 50% male, mean age 26.1 years, evaluated twice over 6 months | Pure-tone and EHF audiometry, otoscopic inspection, immittance and speech audiometry |
| Van Campen et al., 1999b | Longitudinal cohort | 27 survivors of 1995 Oklahoma City bombing who had nonrecorded gaze abnormality or one or more episodes of vertigo or continuing imbalance, mean age 43 years, 50% female and 50% male, evaluated quarterly over 1 year | Balance questionnaire, ENG, CDP |

| Results | Adjustments | Comments or Limitations |
|---------|-------------|-------------------------|
| Side-on incident blast estimated at 3,000 psi at 10 ft to 25 psi at 100 ft.; decibel levels estimated at 235 dB pSPL. 1 year after blast, 76% reported tinnitus, 64% loudness sensitivity, 57% otalgia; averaged across quarters, 76% had mostly sensorineural hearing loss at one or more frequencies; 63% of them were male. 24% required amplification. In CF ranges, males had poorer thresholds than females, but no sex effects for PTA. No clear relationship between location and symptoms or test results. Tympanic perforations healed by second quarter; at 1 year, poorer EHF thresholds in blast subjects with abnormal CF thresholds. | Age-corrected CF | Healthy subjects not age-matched to blast subjects. |
| 60% with abnormal ENG mostly resolved by second quarter; 55% reported nausea with dizziness, 78% tinnitus. At 1 year, 72% said vestibular symptoms were unchanged or occurred intermittently, 67% reported that dizziness was either intermittent or same as first noted, 55% of initially abnormal CDP were normal. Averaged across quarters, SOT showed problems with vestibular (15%), surface-dependent (13%), and physiologically inconsistent (4%) patterns; motor control mostly normal; no relationship between location and tubular symptoms or test results. | | No control group. Timing of postblast health outcome unspecified for several outcome measures. |

*continued*

**TABLE 4-3** Continued

| Reference | Study Design | Population | Health Outcomes or Outcome Measures |
|---|---|---|---|
| Vanderploeg et al., 2012 | Cross-sectional cohort | 1,443 OIF or OEF deployed vs 1,655 nondeployed Florida National Guard; deployed group more likely to be male with some college education and history of psychologic trauma and TBI; subjects assessed an average of 31.8 months after deployment | Web-based survey of symptoms, predeployment trauma or TBI, symptom checklists (including 22-item Neurobehavioral Symptom Inventory), and deployment exposures; blast exposure was categorized as primary and non-primary on the basis of 4 questions |
| Wilk et al., 2012 | Cross-sectional cohort | 3,952 Army OIF service members, 98.3% men, 66.9% less than 30 years old; assessed 3–6 months after deployment | Concussion screening and symptom reporting on Patient Health Questionnaire and question on tinnitus |

NOTES: CDP = computerized dynamic posturography; CF = conventional frequency; CHL = conductive hearing loss; CI = confidence interval; dB pSPL = decibel re: peak sound pressure level; EHF = extended high frequency (10–20 kHz); ENG = electronystagmography; kPa = kilopascal; LOC = loss of consciousness; MHL = mixed hearing loss; NS = nonsignificant; OEF = Operation Enduring Freedom; OIF = Operation Iraqi Freedom; OR = odds ratio; PTA = pure tone audiometry; SNHL = sensorineural hearing loss; SOT = sensory organization test; TBI = traumatic brain injury.

| Results | Adjustments | Comments or Limitations |
|---|---|---|
| 26.3% of deployed reported primary blast, 25.2% reported non-primary blast. Primary blast exposure associated with hearing loss (OR = 2.32; 95% CI, 1.65–3.26; p < 0.001). Non-primary blast exposure associated with hearing loss (OR = 1.63; 95% CI, 1.19–2.24; p < 0.005). Primary blast exposure associated with ringing in ears (OR = 2.92; 95% CI, 2.09–4.09; p < 0.001). Non-primary blast exposure associated with ringing in ears (OR = 1.77; 95% CI, 1.29–2.41; p < 0.005). Primary blast exposure associated with dizziness (OR = 2.26; 95% CI, 1.30–3.94; p < 0.005). Non-primary blast NS for dizziness. | Demographics, predeployment psychologic trauma or TBI and deployment related factors | Low response rate (41.3%) Alpha error rate set at p < 0.01 for multiple comparisons. Assessment of blast injury developed expressly for current study and thus not previously validated. |
| 14.9% met criteria for concussion, 72.2% of whom reported a blast mechanism. Of 201 service members who reported concussion with LOC, blast mechanism was significantly associated with tinnitus compared with nonblast mechanism; no association was found between concussions and change in consciousness. No associations found for dizziness. | | 51.5% response rate. Concussion symptoms self-reported. |

1995. In a cohort study, Shariat et al. (1999) followed up with survivors of the bombing to identify long-term physical and emotional health outcomes. Baseline data on blast exposure and injuries were initially collected after the bombing and recorded in the Injury Prevention Service registry of the Oklahoma State Department of Health. Some 914 survivors of the blast who were 18 years old or older were considered eligible for the study. Of those, 494 (54%) completed a telephone interview that included questions on long-term health conditions, functional status, employment, quality of life, health care use, and medical costs. The followup interview occurred 1.5–3 years after the bombing. The age range of the subjects was 21–91 years (mean = 45 years). Of the subjects, 92% reported being injured in the bombing; 13% sustained injuries that required hospitalization. Of the subjects interviewed, 156 (32%) reported newly diagnosed or treated auditory problems since the bombing. There were significant differences in rates of reports of newly diagnosed auditory problems between those who had been hospitalized and those who had been treated in an emergency department and then released (48% vs 29%; p < 0.006) and between those who had been hospitalized and those who were uninjured or not treated (48% vs 9%, p < 0.001). For tinnitus, 44% of the subjects reported experiencing ringing or roaring in their ears at some time after the bombing, and there was no significant difference between those who had been hospitalized and those who had not. Nearly half the subjects (48%) reported receiving audiology services after the bombing, and there was a significant difference found between those who had been hospitalized and those who were treated and released (72% vs 45%; p = 0.003) or those who were uninjured or not treated (72% vs 29%; p < 0.001). The study has several limitations for the committee's determination of long-term auditory outcomes. For newly diagnosed conditions, it is not clear from the data presented whether the conditions were experienced shortly after the bombing or developed later. At the time of the followup interview, 24% of all newly diagnosed or treated conditions had resolved, but the number of resolved auditory outcomes was not reported. Similarly, at the time of the followup interview, 21% of reported symptoms experienced since the bombing had resolved, but the number of injuries to the auditory system that had resolved was not reported. Other limitations of the study include the low response rate of participation, which could mean that the results reported here are not generalizable to all survivors of the bombing. Measures of tinnitus were based on self-report (no objective measurement is available), and no objective measures of hearing function were analyzed. Self-reporting of "trouble in hearing" and other auditory problems also is a limitation because they are not objective measures.

Van Campen et al. (1999a) conducted a longitudinal cohort study of survivors of the Oklahoma City bombing to examine long-term changes in auditory function. The subject group (83 people) was solicited to participate in the study by advertisements and by referral from physician and personal-assistance programs. Subjects were followed for 1 year during which evaluations, audiometric testing, and a survey questionnaire were completed quarterly. The numbers of subjects present for evaluation and testing at each quarter were 42 0–2 months after the bombing (Q1), 64 3–5 months after the bombing (Q2), 62 6–8 months after the bombing (Q3), and 56 12–14 months after the bombing (Q4). Only 21 (25%) of the subjects were seen at all of the time. Auditory outcomes were compared with those in a representative control group of 10 subjects with normal hearing who were not blast exposed (and not present during the bombing). The control subjects were seen twice over 6 months to document hearing-threshold stability. The results showed no significant differences in pure-tone audiometry (at 1, 2, and 4 kHz) between quarters in either group. Thresholds for high-frequency signals were poorer in blast-exposed persons than in control subjects. At 1 year, use of a hearing aid was recommended for 24% of subjects, none of whom reported hearing aid use before the blast exposure. Tinnitus was reportedly experienced within seconds to days of the blast exposure in 67% of subjects on the Q1 questionnaire. On the Q4 questionnaire, 76% of the responders reported symptoms of tinnitus. There was no clear association between location of subjects in the bombing area and symptoms or test results. Study limitations included the low response rate; only 21 subjects provided responses in each quarter, and the number who were evaluated and questioned in each quarter was variable.

In a companion study, Van Campen et al. (1999b) reported vestibular and balance outcomes in 30 survivors of the Oklahoma City bombing. Subjects were recruited from the sample of 83 included in the previous study, and all were bombing survivors from the downtown area surrounding the blast who reported gaze abnormalities and vertigo or continuing imbalance. The subjects were 25–63 years old (mean, 43 years old). Initially, all subjects completed a questionnaire on their symptoms and underwent nonrecorded gaze testing with computerized dynamic posturography (CDP). The 27 who had abnormal results on the CDP returned quarterly for full balance assessments for a year (Q1, 9 subjects; Q2, 18; Q3, 22; Q4, 24). Thirteen of the 27 (63%) reported dizziness within 48 hours of the explosion. A year after the blast, 16 of 24 (67%) of those assessed at Q4 reported that their symptoms of dizziness and imbalance were unchanged or still intermittent. Results generally showed that testing abnormalities were detected at each quarter, but the data are difficult to interpret because different subjects presented at each testing time; only five subjects were present at all four reporting times over the year. There was no association between subjects' location relative to the blast and their reported symptoms and test results, but 97% of the subjects screened or evaluated in the study were in buildings at the time of the blast. Given that 43% of symptomatic subjects did not report head injury, the vestibular trauma reported may be related to blast overpressure. The study has limitations similar to those of Van Campen et al. (1999a) because of the very small sample and the variability of the followup of subjects (different subjects were evaluated and questioned at each quarter).

Cohen et al. (2002) reported on the auditory and vestibular outcomes of survivors of a terrorist bus bombing in 1994. Of the 48 survivors (18–65 years old; median, 28 years old), 23 were hospitalized; of the 23, 17 continued to be followed for 6 months in an outpatient otolaryngology clinic. Patients underwent otoneurologic examinations and auditory and balance assessments. Results showed that all patients except one had at least one perforated eardrum; there were 27 perforated eardrums. Most (16) of the perforations were considered large, and gradual healing was seen during the followup period. At 6 months, perforations in 15 ears had healed, and perforations in 12 had not healed (possibly because of the number of large perforations). Hearing loss was common; hearing in only one ear was normal immediately after the blast. At 6 months, 6 of the ears had regained normal hearing, for a total of 7 ears with normal hearing. On balance tests, 6 patients had abnormal results and complained of dizziness, and 5 continued to suffer from dizziness throughout the 6 months of followup. At the time of admission to the hospital after the blast, 88% of patients who were followed for 6 months reported aural fullness and pressure; 88%, tinnitus; and 41%, dizziness. At 6 months, 73% of the patients who had reported aural fullness still complained of it, 40% of those who had reported tinnitus still had symptoms of it, and 71% of those who had reported dizziness on admission still had it. The study has limitations for the committee's determination of evidence of long-term auditory outcomes of blast, such as the small sample and the nonmilitary blast exposure. It is unknown whether the findings reported in the study are generalizable to those exposed to blast during military combat. The study also lacked a control group for comparison and did not report outcomes beyond 6 months.

In a retrospective cohort study, Riviere et al. (2008) examined the hearing status of workers who were exposed to an industrial explosion at a chemical plant in France on September 21, 2001. During October 2001– March 2004, all 511 workers underwent audiometric testing, whether or not they were at the site of the explosion. Of the 425 subjects who participated in the study, 208 (49%) had undergone an audiometric test since 1990 but before the explosion. Therefore, the study design made it possible to compare some subjects' pre- and post-blast measures. Subjects were divided into two groups whose outcomes were compared: 103 who were within 1,700 m of the blast and considered "exposed" and 105 who were more than 1,700 m from the blast and therefore considered "less exposed." The average period between preinjury and postinjury audiograms of the exposed group was 1,621 days (SD = ±1,018 days) and for the less exposed group 1,831 days (SD = ±1,121 days). Results comparing pre-blast and post-blast audiograms demonstrated that—with adjustment for age, sex, history of ear problems, and occupational noise exposure—hearing-threshold shifts were greater at 2 and 4 kHz in the right ear in those at shorter distances from the blast. Results from the left ear were different; those at shorter distances had significantly worse threshold shifts at 2, 6, and 8 kHz. In addition, 68% of the exposed group and 46% of the less exposed group had hearing loss of 10 dB or more affecting at least one ear at 2, 4, or 6 kHz (p < 0.01). The study design made it possible to compare pre-blast audiometric measures between an exposed group and a less exposed group. However, the study did not control for confounding factors, such as other exposures that may cause hearing loss. And although some subjects had followup testing more than 2 years after injury, other subjects had followup testing as little as a month after the exposure, and their results are therefore short-term results. The data were not analyzed to examine changes in hearing loss over time after the explosion.

Vanderploeg et al. (2012) conducted a cross-sectional cohort study by using data collected in anonymous online surveys to determine whether there was an association between military experience and immediate and long-term physical and psychologic health outcomes. The study also aimed to examine the effects of multiple deployment-related TBIs on health outcomes. About 10,400 letters were mailed to members of the Florida National Guard to invite participation in the survey; 4,005 people (41.3%) completed the survey, and those who had been deployed completed it an average of 31.8 months (SD = 24.4 months, range = 0–95 months) after their deployment; 3,098 subjects (1,443 who had deployed and 1,655 who had not deployed) were included in the study. ORs were calculated to assess the association between current health status and deployment-related factors, such as physical injuries, exposure to potentially traumatic deployment experiences, combat, blast exposure, and mild TBI. Demographics and predeployment experiences were controlled for as potential confounders. Many questions were included on the survey to measure predictors of health outcomes, including blast exposure. Of the 3,098 subjects in the study sample, 24% reported having been exposed to blast, but 51% of those who had deployed reported having been so exposed. Results showed a statistically significant difference in reported hearing loss between deployed subjects and non-deployed subjects (29% vs 9%, p < 0.001) and a statistically significant difference in reported tinnitus (32% vs 10%, respectively, p < 0.001). Subjects who had been exposed to blast had higher odds of hearing loss (AOR = 1.63 [95% CI, 1.59–6.65] after nonprimary blast exposure and 2.32 [95% CI, 1.65–3.26] after primary blast exposure), tinnitus (AOR = 1.77 [95% CI, 1.29–2.41] for nonprimary blast exposure and 2.92 [95% CI, 2.09, 4.09] for primary blast exposure), and dizziness (AOR = 2.26 [95% CI, 1.30–3.94] primary blast exposure only). The limitations of the study include a low response rate (41%), which limits the generalizability of the results to all deployed or non-deployed service members, and lack of information about other possible exposures that may have caused injury during deployment or led to auditory problems. The study also relied on self-reported measures for all outcomes and did not include any objective measures or test results.

Wilk et al. (2012) conducted a survey of three infantry brigades 3–6 months after their return from deployment to determine the extent to which a screening for blast concussion identifies people who are at higher risk for persistent postconcussive symptoms. The survey included questions about physical symptoms (including questions about auditory and vestibular symptoms), postconcussive symptoms, and mental health conditions. Of the 7,668 service members in the three brigades, 4,383 (57%) consented and completed part of the survey, and 3,952 (52%) completed the concussion questions. Most who did not participate were on leave or unavailable because of duty assignments (more than 93% of service members who attended the briefings about the study agreed to participate). Results showed that 201 people had had a concussion with LOC, 161 of whom had had a blast-related concussion. Service members who had had a blast concussion reported more tinnitus than those who had had non-blast concussion (34% vs 15%, p = 0.02). However, there was no association between blast concussion and dizziness. A limitation of the study is the subjective quality of the data, which are based exclusively on self-report. In addition, the small number of service members reporting symptoms limits the power of statistical comparisons.

## Supportive Studies

Supportive studies identified by the committee have important limitations. Many had small sample or selection biases and covered only short-term followup. And many of the studies used self-report measures and self-reports of exposure to blast, so they lack objective data. St. Onge et al. (2011) was the only secondary study that used pre-blast measures. The study aimed to understand auditory and vestibular outcomes in marines enrolled in the Breacher Training Course, which includes exposure to blast explosions. Pure-tone hearing thresholds were collected before and after the training of 38 marines. Results showed significantly worse thresholds after exposure at 1, 2, and 3 kHz. Generally, the study found that hearing loss was statistically and clinically significant, whereas vestibular findings were not significant. It used short-term followup and was not meant to study the long-term auditory and vestibular effects of the Breacher Training Course, so it does not contribute to determination of long-term outcomes of exposure to blast.

In a retrospective chart review, Lew et al. (2011) examined 36,426 patient records in the DOD Defense Manpower Data Center to determine the prevalence of self-reported auditory, visual, and dual sensory impairment in Afghanistan and Iraq war veterans who received TBI evaluations. All 12,521 subjects included in the study had screened positive in an initial TBI evaluation and then had a comprehensive second-level TBI evaluation. As part of the second-level examination, measures of self-reported blast exposure and sensory symptoms, including hearing difficulty, were collected. The subjects were compared with a control group of 9,106 who had no reported TBI. For auditory impairment, there was a significant association between history of blast exposure and severity of sensory complaint [$\chi^2$ (3) = 198.20, p < 0.0001; Cramer's V = 0.13]. Specifically, a higher percentage of blast-exposed TBI patients than of non-blast-exposed TBI patients reported moderate to very severe impairment. Although the study had an adequate sample size, data on blast exposure were based on self-reports. In addition, although the study is analytically sophisticated, it provides a conditional analysis that is based on those who have TBI and then models the contribution of blast to self-reported sensory impairment. For example, given the presence of TBI, what is the effect of blast exposure?

### Additional Long-Term Effects of Blast Injury on Auditory Function

Hearing loss as measured by increased pure-tone thresholds is an immediate and long-term effect of blast exposure and is probably due to blast-related damage to the auditory periphery (middle-ear and inner-ear structures). The changes may present as complaints related to loss of hearing acuity (that is, the ability to hear low-level sounds). With the healing of middle-ear structures and recovery of cochlear function, hearing thresholds may return to pre-blast values. However, injuries due to blast exposure can also involve the central auditory nervous system and affect accurate supra-threshold processing of the spectral and temporal properties of sounds in three-dimensional space (Gallun et al., 2012a,b; Valiyaveettil et al., 2012). Such changes may present as complaints of difficulty in conversing or localizing sound in noisy environments even though sounds are clearly audible. Precise binaural encoding of sound patterns is required for understanding speech, appreciating music, recognizing environmental sounds, and localizing sound in complex environments that have background noise, reverberation, and multiple talkers originating in different sound sources. Impairments may persist even when post-blast hearing thresholds are normal or have returned to normal, as measured by conventional audiometry.

Although the study of central auditory dysfunction in maintaining normal communication and complex sound processing is advancing, the sites of injury and underlying mechanisms responsible for specific symptoms are not known. Therefore, standardized clinical test batteries to assess the functions are not available, and there is no consensus on appropriate treatment for the communication deficits. Moreover, there is only sparse evidence on auditory effects of multiple blast exposures, medication use, and comorbid conditions, such as mild TBI and other brain injuries, PTSD, multisensory impairments, and cognitive losses related to attention and memory.

## Conclusions

Blast can injure the auditory system both acutely and over the long term. There is a consensus that blast can cause perforation of the tympanic membrane and disruption of the ossicular chain and result in conductive hearing loss, which may be permanent or resolve with treatment or the spontaneous closure of the TM. The evidence needed to determine the likelihood of long-term hearing loss through this mechanism is lacking. It is common to experience an immediate loss of hearing sensitivity after blast exposure, which may not be associated with TM rupture or middle-ear damage. That loss of hearing may reflect cochlear damage from the noise exposure and improve with time; again, the literature is not adequate to estimate the risk of long-term hearing loss. Blast exposure may also affect the auditory system through inflammation, effects on microcirculation, brain edema, ototoxic side effects of medications given for other injuries, and many other mechanisms, but there is no consensus on the long-term consequences. Similarly, with respect to recurrent blast exposure that leads to cumulative changes in structure at the microscopic level, there is no consensus on whether it has long-term consequences. It is possible that blast causes dysfunction in dimensions of auditory function beyond declines in hearing acuity, which may go undetected or unnoticed in the immediate period after exposure, and there is no consensus on whether this dysfunction has long-term consequences and how long changes in auditory processing abilities may persist after hearing thresholds return to pre-blast values. Finally, there are no data with which it can be determined whether blast-related injuries increase the risk of age-related changes in hearing acuity (presbycusis) or suprathreshold auditory processing or accelerate the aging process and result in early onset of these conditions.

> The committee concludes, on the basis of its evaluation, that there is limited/suggestive evidence of an association between exposure to blast and long-term effects on the tympanic membrane and auditory thresholds.

The committee concludes, on the basis of its evaluation, that there is inadequate/insufficient evidence of an association between exposure to blast and tinnitus and long-term effects on central auditory processing.

The committee concludes, on the basis of its evaluation, that there is inadequate/insufficient evidence of an association between exposure to blast and long-term balance dysfunction and vertigo.

## OCULAR OUTCOMES

Exposure to blast can lead to severe eye injuries, often from debris that hits the eyes and leads to blunt or penetrating injuries. Signs of ocular blast injury include bleeding, preorbital swelling or bruising, 360-degree conjunctival hemorrhage, misshapen pupil, pigmented or clear gel-like tissue outside the globe, and an abnormal shape of the anterior chamber. Symptoms are wide-ranging and include minimal discomfort, foreign body sensation, severe pain, and decreased, altered, or total loss of vision. It is important to note that there can be serious damage to the eye in the absence of vision loss or serious signs and symptoms, especially with nonpenetrating injuries.

### Acute and Well-Known Long-Term Effects

Serious open-globe injuries in the form of laceration and rupture occur in 20–50% of those who have blast eye injuries (Morley et al., 2010; Peral Gutierrez De Ceballos et al., 2005; Tucker and Lettin, 1975). Such injuries are predominantly secondary blast injuries from sharp propelled particles that cause penetration, perforation, and the implantation of intraocular foreign bodies. Choroidal rupture also is possible from blunt trauma or blast wave but is less likely (Alam et al., 2012). Closed-globe injuries to the eye can result in small corneal abrasions, conjunctivitis, and superficial foreign bodies; these outcomes typically would occur when debris makes contact with the surface of the eye in a secondary blast injury. However, more serious outcomes from closed globe injuries are possible too—mainly from blunt trauma and primary blast injury (PBI)—and include hyphema, vitreous hemorrhage, commotio retinae, retinal detachment, macular holes, traumatic cataract, optic nerve damage, and orbital fracture (Alam et al., 2012; Morley et al., 2010). Blast injuries, particularly open-globe injuries, may result in loss of an eye, permanent blindness, or vision impairment.

The visual system requires more than an intact eye free of important pathology for normal function, as the information encoded by the retina must be correctly and efficiently transmitted to the visual cortex for processing and integration. In addition to overt ocular injuries, damage to the visual system caused by blast may disrupt these neural networks. Near vision (reading) problems, light sensitivity, accommodative insufficiency, and convergence insufficiency have been reported in blast-injured patients (Magone et al., 2013). Similar visual symptoms can occur following a mild TBI.

## Additional Long-Term Effects

To evaluate the long-term ocular health effects of blast exposure, the committee reviewed about 75 published peer-reviewed studies. No available studies met enough of the inclusion guidelines to be considered primary. This section details the identified supportive studies on long-term ocular health outcomes of blast exposure.

Goodrich et al. (2007), in a retrospective descriptive study, conducted a record review of patients seen in the Optometry Polytrauma Inpatient Clinic (OPTIC) at the VA Palo Alto Health Care System during December 2004–November 2006. The study aimed to assess visual function in patients who experienced deployment-related polytrauma. Data examined in the study were derived from OPTIC's extensive examination protocol, which includes self-report questions about vision status before and after the injury, clinical measurements of distance and near visual acuity, visual fields, binocular-vision status, and other vision measures. The study compared 25 who had blast-related injuries with 25 who had other than blast injuries and found a higher rate of visual injury in the blast-injured group (13 vs 5). Blasts resulted in penetrating head injuries in 11 cases and all other causes produced penetrating head injuries in four cases. All four people who had total blindness, clearly a long-term effect, had blast-related injuries. Although this study provided good vision-examination data in addition to self-reported vision data on blast-injured patients, for several reasons it has only limited usefulness for establishing evidence of long-term ocular outcomes of blast. First, it had a small selected sample that was biased in that the subjects were patients in a polytrauma center who stayed long enough to be examined (that is, had severe injuries), and all had TBI; therefore, the results may not be generalizable to the larger population of those who suffer minor injuries from exposure to blast or those who do not have TBI. In addition, there was no statistical analysis of the differences in visual problems between blast-injured and non-blast-injured groups, and analyses did not control for confounding. In a followup study, Goodrich et al. (2013) conducted statistical analysis of group differences in ocular outcomes between the two groups from the 2007 study (blast-related and non-blast-injured); the analysis found few significant differences in visual dysfunction between the two groups.

Brahm et al. (2009) conducted another retrospective study that analyzed data from electronic examination records of vision screenings completed in the VA Palo Alto Health Care System. Screening results were examined for 68 consecutive patients (57 were blast-injured) who were evaluated in the VA Polytrauma Rehabilitation Center (PRC) during August 2006–December 2007 and 124 consecutive patients (112 were blast-injured) who were evaluated in the VA Polytrauma Network Site (PNS) clinic during August 2006–December 2007. The patients evaluated in the PRC were seen for inpatient care and had moderate to severe TBI. Those evaluated in the PNS clinic were seen on an outpatient basis, had no life-threatening injuries, and had screened positive for mild TBI. The frequency of ocular injury, visual impairment, and visual dysfunction was examined in the two groups, and differences between blast-injured and non-blast-injured were described. The results were inconsistent in the inpatient and outpatient groups with regard to visual dysfunction and blast injury. In the inpatient group, the blast-injured were more likely to have ocular injuries than the non-blast-injured; in the outpatient group, the blast-injured were less likely to have ocular injuries than the non-blast-injured. The rate of moderate visual-acuity loss was higher in the blast-injured patients than in the non-blast-injured in the inpatient group (20 of 70 and 20 of 100) and such loss was too rare in the outpatient group to support useful conclusions. This study has limitations similar to those of Goodrich et al. (2007) in having a biased sample of only polytrauma inpatients and outpatients and no control groups. In addition, there was no statistical analysis of between-group differences in blast-injured and non-blast-injured patients. Another limitation is the lack of objective measure of blast exposure, although the study did have reasonable measures of visual dysfunction. Because the study was retrospective and did not control for confounding variables, it is impossible to determine the associated risk of visual dysfunction due specifically to blast exposure.

Coe et al. (2010) conducted a prospective study that followed combat-injured service members seen in the ophthalmology service of WRAMC during September 2003–February 2005. All 11 patients in the study had eye injuries and retained corneal foreign bodies secondary to blast trauma. They were compared with age-matched and sex-matched uninjured controls. There were numerous inclusion and exclusion criteria (for example, no other penetrating injuries and no concurrent inflammation or infection), and patients were excluded for any physical or mental impairment that would prevent them from undergoing eye examinations or providing informed consent for the study. Followup time was 1–6 months. Results showed no statistically significant differences in visual acuity with high contrast, but visual performance of injured eyes was significantly worse than that of control eyes on photopic low-contrast visual acuity ($p < 0.001$), mesopic low-contrast visual acuity without glare ($p < 0.001$), mesopic low-contrast visual acuity with glare ($p = 0.0007$), and contrast sensitivity (p < 0.0001). The study has limitations; the small sample and sample selection bias in which extensive inclusion and exclusion criteria were used (those with complex eye injuries were excluded from the study sample). The results may therefore not be generalizable to the larger population of blast-exposed people. In addition, the statistical analyses did not control for potential confounders, and the followup period was short.

In a retrospective chart review Lew et al. (2011) examined 36,426 patient records in the Defense Manpower Data Center to determine the prevalence of self-reported auditory, visual, and dual sensory impairment in Afghanistan and Iraq war veterans who were evaluated for TBI. All 12,521 subjects included in the study had screened positive in an initial TBI evaluation and then had a comprehensive second-level TBI evaluation. As part of the second-level examination, measures of self-reported blast exposure and sensory symptoms were collected, including vision problems (blurring and trouble in seeing) and hearing difficulty. The subjects were compared with a control group of 9,106 who had no reported TBI (although the number of TBI cases may have been underreported). In a multiple linear regression model for visual impairment, blast exposure accounted for 0.14% of the variance. Other factors that accounted for variance were age (1.1%), sex (0.5%), auditory impairment (9.3%), and TBI (0.69%). Although the study had an adequate sample size, it reported only limited data on blast exposure. In addition, although the study was analytically sophisticated, it provided a conditional analysis based on those who have TBI and on modeling of the contribution of blast to self-reported visual impairment (for example, given the presence of TBI, what is the effect of blast exposure?).

In a case control study, Scheibel et al. (2012) examined service members and veterans to compare functional outcomes between those who had TBI and blast exposure and in those who did not. The study included 15 subjects who screened positive for TBI (all with at least one blast exposure) and 15 controls who had been similarly deployed but with no blast exposure or TBI. Results of fMRI demonstrated that the TBI group had increased activation in areas involved in visual perception, attention, and visuo-spatial functions (anterior cingulate gyrus, medial frontal cortex, and posterior cerebral areas). The study also attempted to evaluate other differences between cases and controls and reported that there were no major differences in self-reported alcohol or other drug use, psychiatric symptoms, or medication use. The study has limitations due to the biased sample of cases, 13 of which came from a TBI clinic at one VA medical center. In addition, the control group was not matched for combat exposure. With respect to understanding visual outcomes of blast exposure, the study is limited in that no direct measures of vision were used; instead, the study examined brain imaging results to quantify activation differences in visual perception between the two groups.

Capo-Aponte et al. (2012) examined the occurrence of visual dysfunction in 20 subjects who received care at WRAMC and had suffered blast-induced mild TBI within the preceding 45 days (median time between blast exposure and evaluation, 30.5 days; range, 16–45 days). A control group of 20 age-matched subjects was recruited and evaluated at the US Army Aeromedical Research Lab in Rucker, Alabama. The controls had been deployed but had no history of TBI, head concussion, or blast exposure. Results showed no statistical differences in manifest refraction and intraocular pressure between the two groups. Oculomotor function tests demonstrated that the mild-TBI group had more defective eye movements than the control group, but there was no significant difference in fixation disparity and flat fusion. The mild-TBI group had worse reading speed (p = 0.0019) and reading comprehension scores (p = 0.0106) and more reports of light sensitivity, eye strain, and reading-associated symptoms. The study has limitations due to the small sample size, and the sample may also have been biased in that case subjects were selected from a single medical center. In addition, the controls were healthy subjects whereas the cases were receiving treatment in a medical center, so between-group differences associated with blast may be overestimated. For the purposes of the committee's review of possible long-term ocular outcomes of blast exposure, the study is limited in its usefulness owing to the short-term followup and the lack of data on longer-term outcomes. The study did document clinician records of symptoms experienced by patients.

The committee determined that 40 additional studies met the guidelines for inclusion in the committee's review as tertiary but had little usefulness in demonstrating evidence on the long-term ocular health effects of blast exposure. The two studies that were the most useful for the committee's review are discussed below.

Cockerham et al. (2013) conducted a prospective observational cohort study of patients who had TBI and were receiving care at a PRC from 2010 to 2012. Blast exposure was the mechanism of injury of 44 of the 53 subjects. The subjects were compared with an age-matched and sex-matched control group of 18 healthy subjects. The study provided long-term followup of some of the patients in the Goodrich et al. (2007) study described above. The reported time since injury ranged from 1 to 60 months, with a median of 6 months. Results showed that the TBI group had significantly more dry-eye disease symptoms than the control group. With respect to objective measures, 93% of the TBI group had at least one test result indicative of dry-eye disease compared with 44% of the control group ($\chi^2$ = 19.56; p < 0.001). Prevalence of abnormal dry-eye test results was generally similar in the subjects who had TBI caused by blast and those who had TBI not caused by blast. However, for the measure of tear-film breakup time, none of the non-blast TBI subjects and 33% of the blast TBI subjects had values below 10 seconds. That difference was just short of statistical significance ($\chi^2 = 3.2$; $p = 0.07$). The study also found no relationship between use of particular medications (presumed to have an effect on eye function) and dry-eye disease measures. The study has limitations owing to its small sample and typical selection bias in that the TBI cases were all from one polytrauma center and probably severely injured, whereas the controls were healthy. That bias may have led to larger observed differences between cases and controls. In addition, the study authors do not specify whether blast exposure was controlled for but noted that the controls did not have TBI.

In a retrospective consecutive-case series, Blanch et al. (2011) reported injury patterns and long-term outcomes of eye injuries sustained from July 2004 through May 2008 by British armed forces personnel who were deployed to Iraq and Afghanistan. Mean followup of those who had closed-globe injuries was 245 days, and that of those who had open-globe injuries was 220 days. The assessed ocular outcomes reported in the study include final best-corrected visual acuity, rates of endophthalmitis, and proliferative vitreoretinopathy. Of the 630 people who had major traumatic injury, 63 (10%) suffered ocular injuries. Of 34 eyes with initial visual acuity ≤6/60, 18 had final visual acuity <6/60. A total of 17 eyes had a final visual acuity of 1/60 or worse, of which 6 were in three patients (bilateral). The causes were rupture or extensive disruption (nine eyes), corneal scar (two eyes), proliferative vitreoretinopathy (two eyes), traumatic optic neuropathy (one eye), subfoveal choroidal rupture (one eye), intraocular foreign-body-impacted fovea (one eye), and retinal burns from hot intraocular foreign body (one eye). Of the 56 subjects not recorded as wearing eye protection, 11 had poor visual outcomes (they could not see hand movements or worse) compared with one of the seven who wore eye protection. Although the study did not compare ocular outcomes by mechanism of injury, explosive blast injuries occurred in 54 of the 63 (86%). The study has limitations for the committee's review of long-term ocular outcomes of blast, mainly in the case-series study design. Without a control group and without comparison of blast with non-blast injuries, it is unknown what amount and type of ocular injury is attributable specifically to blast.

## Conclusions

Blast can cause both acute and long-term serious ocular injuries. Permanent ocular symptoms and structural alterations can occur in isolation or in conjunction with TBI. There is a consensus that blast can cause structural alterations that lead to long-term effects on ocular function. The structures most commonly associated with substantial visual loss are the cornea, the retina, and the optic nerve. The injuries typically need to be bilateral to affect long-term afferent function (that is, ability to read or drive). In contrast, damage to the efferent system by definition creates a bilateral issue of dysmotility, including issues of fixation stability, diplopia, vergence, and fusion.

There is no consensus as to whether blast exposure that causes no visible change in structure but does cause symptoms has long-term consequences. The most common symptoms reported are photophobia, eyestrain, and headache.

The long-term implications of blast injury when there are known objective measures of subclinical injury are poorly understood. The implications include tear production and stability, endothelial cell count, ganglion cell loss, and fMRI alterations in the regions of the brain involved in visual function.

Finally, there are no data to determine whether blast-related ocular injuries increase the risk of such age-related conditions as cataract or macular degeneration or of early onset of presbyopia, loss of contrast sensitivity, or other visual abnormalities.

> The committee concludes, on the basis of its evaluation, that there is sufficient evidence of a causal relationship between penetrating eye injuries resulting from exposure to blast and permanent blindness and visual impairment (visual acuity of 20/40 or worse).

> The committee concludes, on the basis of its evaluation, that there is inadequate/insufficient evidence of an association between exposure to blast that leads to acute nonpenetrating eye injuries and long-term effects on vision.

## CARDIOVASCULAR OUTCOMES

For the purposes of this report, cardiovascular outcomes are defined as myocardial conditions, all vascular conditions, and cardiovascular death.

### Acute Effects

Cardiovascular injury in blast victims can occur through many mechanisms and usually has the potential for severe and even fatal outcomes even if treatment is timely. The most severe outcome, cardiorespiratory arrest, occurs in 1–4% of all trauma patients (Tarmey et al., 2011). Blast injury to the cardiovascular system can be caused by the blast wave, penetrating projectiles, and blunt trauma (primary, secondary, tertiary, and quaternary blast injury). It can occur from direct damage to the thorax or appendages, it can result from blast injuries to other organ systems, and blast injury to any part of the body can lead to vascular damage.

The main mechanisms of direct vascular injury caused by a blast are avulsion, perforation, and laceration of major vessels in extremities and the neck, mostly due to secondary—but also tertiary and quaternary—blast injury (Fasol et al., 1989). The two immediate outcomes of these injuries are exsanguination and ischemia. Loss of pulse occurs rapidly with exsanguination, and victims will have a poor prognosis, often death (Tarmey et al., 2011). Ischemia will result in tissue death if blood supply to deprived areas is not restored quickly, and amputation will need to be performed (Barros D'Sa et al., 1980; Fasol et al., 1989). Vascular injuries secondary to blast injuries may not be readily apparent at the time of the initial blast. The recognition that those vascular lesions can be occult has clear implications for long-term outcomes because they would be expected to be severe if vascular lesions are not immediately identified.

Direct cardiac injury to the thorax can be primary, secondary, tertiary, and quaternary blast injury and can cause myocardial contusions, arterial air emboli, valvular and cardiac-chamber rupture, pericardial injury and tamponade, conduction abnormalities, and cardiac rhythm irregularities (arrythmias) (Mayorga, 1997; Ozer et al., 2009). The more severe of those conditions, such as cardiac-chamber damage, result from the rare occurrence of tears or lacerations of the myocardium after high blast overpressure (Mayorga, 1997).

Blast trauma directly or indirectly affecting the cardiovascular system commonly causes arrhythmias. The arrythmias include bradycardia, which can eventually progress to asystole (Mayorga, 1997; Ritenour and Baskin, 2008), and various tachycardias, including such fatal forms as ventricular fibrillation. That blast trauma may induce abnormalities and dysfunction in the autonomic nervous system has potential long-term implications for cardiovascular health. Blast victims may have other hemodynamic effects that change blood concentrations and function. Acute coagulopathy, an impairment of the blood's ability to clot, often arises with traumatic injury. Simmons et al. (2011) showed that patients injured by explosions were more coagulopathic than those who suffered gunshot wounds. Cervical dissection and carotid–cavernous fistulas associated with blast-induced craniofacial trauma and TBI have been reported (Vadivelu et al., 2010). These types of injuries may be subject to delayed presentation and detection. Diastolic hypertension was reported in persons hospitalized after an explosion in Texas in 1947 (Ruskin et al., 1948); in most cases, the patients' blood pressure returned to normal within a few months of the explosion (Ruskin and Beard, 1948).

Additional cardiovascular effects may develop quickly from blast injuries to other organ systems. For example, air emboli that develop from damaged lungs at alveolar–pulmonary venous fistulae can cause myocardial ischemia or infarction and are thought to pose the most immediate threat to life in blast victims (Mayorga, 1997; Phillips, 1986). Another example is the release of potentially toxic muscle cell components and electrolytes into the bloodstream that can occur with a crush injury (CDC, 2010).

## Long-Term Effects

The committee considered 31 relevant studies to determine long-term cardiovascular effects of blast exposure. None of them met the committee's inclusion guidelines for primary studies. None reported on actual long-term (longer than 6 months) cardiovascular health effects of blast, so the committee had sparse information on which to base conclusions. This section summarizes the small number of supportive studies, which may begin to inform understanding of possible long-term cardiovascular health outcomes of blast exposure.

The study of most usefulness for the committee's review of long-term cardiovascular effects was Johnson et al. (2007b), a case-series study designed to analyze the sensitivity and specificity of physical examinations to detect vascular lesions after combat-related extremity wounds. The study found that physical examination was not a reliable means of excluding occult or delayed posttraumatic arterial lesions. Compared with arteriography, physical examination had a positive predictive value of about 85% and a negative predictive value of only 50%. For proximal injuries, physical examination had worse reliability, with a positive predictive value of 15% and a negative predictive value of 60%. However, the study has major limitations in its usefulness for the committee's review of long-term cardiovascular outcomes of blast exposure. Of the 99 patients included in the study, although 82% had primary blast- or explosion-related injuries, there was no comparison of blast-exposed with non-blast-exposed patients. In addition, possible delayed effects of the combat-related extremity wounds were evaluated 2–14 days after injury, so the usefulness of this study in understanding long-term cardiovascular outcomes is limited.

No other studies provided the committee with evidence of possible long-term cardiovascular health outcomes of blast, but some supportive studies helped to inform the committee's assessment. Tarmey et al. (2011) was a case-series study of 52 patients who had traumatic cardiopulmonary arrest and were admitted to a military trauma center in Afghanistan; the principal mechanism of injury was IEDs. Lower limbs were the most common sites of injury, and exsanguination was the most common cause of arrest in the patients. The study tracked the patients through hospital discharge; of the 52 included in the study, only four survived to discharge. The study reported that all four had good neurologic recovery, but long-term cardiovascular outcomes after arrest were not reported. The study is limited in its usefulness for the committee's review because there was no long-term followup of the survivors. In addition, there was no control group, nor was a specific population defined as blast-injured. The study is informative as to the likelihood of survival (poor but comparable with rates in other studies) of patients who had traumatic cardiopulmonary arrest and were victims of IEDs. Hilz et al. (2011) reported on long-term (5- to 43-month) cardiovascular outcomes after mild TBI and found that mild-TBI patients had less cardiovagal modulation and baroreflex sensitivity while supine than did a health control group. On standing, the mild-TBI patients still had reduced baroreflex sensitivity and did not withdraw parasympathetic or augment sympathetic modulation adequately. Although this study suggests that impaired autonomic modulation probably contributes to cardiovascular irregularities after mild TBI, the mechanism of the initial TBI was not reported, so the study does not address whether these effects would be seen in a population exposed specifically to blast.

The association between cardiovascular disease and war-related amputations has been recognized since World War II (Hrubec and Ryder, 1980). In a study of 3,890 World War II survivors who had proximal limb amputations and were followed for more than 30 years, the relative risks of total and cardiovascular mortality were 2.4 and 4.0, respectively. In those who had distal amputations, the relative risks of total and cardiovascular mortality were 1.44 and 1.45. Mechanisms by which amputation may lead to future cardiovascular disease include lack of physical activity, which leads to weight gain and obesity, and increased coagulability.

## Conclusions

The committee identified no literature that assessed direct long-term effects of blast injuries on cardiovascular health. Long-term cardiovascular outcomes of blast exposure have not been studied specifically, but the committee deduced that long-term effects may be likely in patients who have severe traumatic limb injuries. The committee found that in patients who had severe traumatic limb injuries, there was a high proportion of occult vascular lesions, including arteriovenous fistulas and aneurysms. Some of those clinically silent lesions require interventions. On the basis of prior knowledge, these lesions can be said to have long-term health consequences for the limb and generally for the vascular system.

**The committee concludes, on the basis of its evaluation, that there is limited/suggestive evidence of an association between major limb injuries, including amputations, resulting from exposure to blast and long-term outcomes for the affected limb and for the cardiac system.**

The committee concludes, on the basis of its evaluation, that there is inadequate/insufficient evidence of an association between exposure to blast and long-term effects on cardiovascular function, such as accelerated atherosclerosis.

## RESPIRATORY OUTCOMES

Exposure to blast can affect both the upper respiratory tract (the nose, the nasal cavity, paranasal sinuses, the pharynx, and the larynx) and the lower respiratory tract (the trachea, the bronchi, the bronchioles, and the alveoli). The discussion that follows focuses on the lower respiratory tract (the lungs). Other parts of the respiratory tract are susceptible to burns that result from blast; such burns are discussed later in this chapter.

### Acute Effects

Blast lung injury (BLI) is the second most frequent injury in blast survivors and the most common fatal primary blast injury in initial survivors of an explosion (Finlay et al., 2012; IOM, 2009). BLI occurs when a blast wave affects the chest cavity and creates overpressure that causes alveolar contusion, tearing, and stripping of the airway epithelium (Avidan et al., 2005; CDC, 2012; Cooper et al., 1983). Contusion of the lung, in the absence of other complications, is the less severe of the acute outcomes and usually develops and resolves within a week of the exposure. Tearing of the alveolar tissue and airway epithelial damage cause hemorrhage, edema, and fistula and can lead to more serious conditions, such as hemothorax, pneumothorax, and air emboli (Argyros, 1997; Avidan et al., 2005; CDC, 2012; Cooper et al., 1983). Patients who have BLI typically present with dyspnea, chest pain, trouble in breathing, coughing, hypoxia, and respiratory following a characteristic latent period that can extend up to 48 hours after the explosion.

There are several less common acute effects of blast exposure on the lungs. Secondary, tertiary, and quaternary blast injuries to the chest—propelled shrapnel, body displacement into a fixed object, and structural collapse, respectively—can cause blunt trauma and, less commonly, penetrating damage (Caseby and Porter, 1976). Blunt trauma to the chest is pathologically similar to BLI; pulmonary contusion is the most prominent outcome. The defining difference between BLI and blunt trauma to the lung is that the latter has a much lower likelihood and severity of alveolar tear and fistula (Caseby and Porter, 1976). Burn injuries to the upper respiratory tract are not uncommon in the Iraq and Afghanistan wars and may occur from inhalation of hot air in connection with blast exposure (Eckert et al., 2006). Thermal injuries to the respiratory system are classified as quaternary blast injuries and can have unpredictable outcomes, including permanent fibrosis of the bronchial mucosa (Krzywiecki et al., 2007).

Beyond the traditional enumeration of blast injuries, blast lung and other severe blast injuries necessitate critical care. Patients might be presumed to be at risk for the common complications of critical illness, including ventilator-associated pneumonia, line infections, and weakness acquired in the setting of an intensive care unit (ICU). Complications also can include cognitive and psychologic disorders (Desai et al., 2011; Needham et al., 2012; Schweickert and Hall, 2007). Those problems have been shown to lead to substantial new disability and cognitive impairments in patients who have severe sepsis and general critical illness (Cuthbertson et al., 2010; Herridge et al., 2011; Iwashyna et al., 2010)—sometimes termed post-intensive-care syndrome (PICS) (Needham et al., 2012)—but have not themselves been studied in survivors of BLI.

## Long-Term Effects

To evaluate the long-term respiratory health effects of blast exposure, the committee reviewed about 45 published peer-reviewed studies. No available studies met enough of the inclusion guidelines to be considered primary. This section details the identified supportive studies on long-term respiratory health outcomes of blast exposure.

Two secondary studies examined the long-term respiratory outcomes of acute BLI. In a case-series study, Hirshberg et al. (1999) examined long-term lung function in 11 people who survived acute BLI after terrorist bus attacks in Jerusalem in 1996. Ten of the 11 required mechanical ventilation and ICU support. One year after injury, lung-function tests were completed on all 11 survivors; results were normal in 9, and none of the 11 had pulmonary complaints. Those findings of a small study suggest that patients follow a trajectory of complete recovery with regard to lung function; other nonpulmonary sequelae of their blast injury were not reported. The study had limitations due to the small number of subjects. In a retrospective case series, Avidan et al. (2005) looked at the long-term respiratory health outcomes in victims of terrorist bombing attacks who sustained acute BLI and survived an ICU admission during December 1983–February 2004 in a single hospital in Israel. Of the 29 patients eligible for inclusion in the study, 76% required mechanical ventilation. Of the 29, 28 survived to the time of the followup interview, 21 (75%) of whom responded to the interview and reported on their long-term outcomes. Of the 21, 16 (76%) reported no respiratory handicap, required no respiratory therapy, and were free of symptoms; the remaining 5 (24%) reported respiratory symptoms and some degree of respiratory dysfunction, but two of them had a history of asthma dating to before the blast exposure. The study showed no consistent pattern of association between blast exposure and long-term respiratory health outcomes and lacks the clinical granularity needed to evaluate the likely trajectories of participants. Like the Hirshberg et al. (1999) study, this one was limited by its small sample and lack of a control group. The followup period was longer (6 months to 21 years), but it was limited by variable followup and the use of self-reports of symptoms gathered through telephone interviews.

Two other studies provided further information on possible long-term respiratory outcomes of a blast explosion. In a retrospective cohort study, Krzywiecki et al. (2007) reported on miners who were exposed to a methane explosion and sustained thermal injury. The study included a control group of healthy miners who had a similar period of work underground and were not exposed to the methane explosion. Long-term lung function was measured at baseline (5–7 months after the explosion) and then 6 years later. At baseline, there was no significant difference in mean pulmonary function tests (PFTs) between the exposed miners and the control group. After 6 years, PFTs showed a significantly lower ($p < 0.01$) forced expiratory volume in 1 second in exposed miners than in the control group. Mean absolute decreases in functional tests did not differ significantly between the exposed and control groups, except that diffusing capacity decreased more in the exposed miners and the maximal expiratory flow at 50% of vital flow capacity decreased more in the control group. The study is limited in that the exposure was not only to blast but to heat and carbon monoxide. Furthermore, the study did not adjust for different rates of smoking and different age groups between the exposed and control groups.

The final secondary study examined long-term pulmonary function after severe blunt chest trauma (Kishikawa et al., 1991). It was a case-series study that examined two groups of patients prospectively. One group had followup 6 months after injury, and some had pulmonary contusion. The other group had followup 1–4 years after injury, and all had an initial diagnosis of pulmonary contusion. Generally, patients in each group who had a diagnosis of pulmonary contusion performed worse in PFTs. The study had limited usefulness for the committee's review because the mechanism of injury was blunt chest trauma, not specifically blast exposure. In addition, the study had a small number of subjects and no matched control group. However, the study is informative inasmuch as pulmonary contusion is a possible acute outcome of blast exposure, and it showed a difference in lung function over the long term between those who had pulmonary contusions and those who did not.

The committee determined that three additional studies met the guidelines for inclusion in its review as tertiary but had limited usefulness in presenting evidence on the long-term respiratory health effects of blast exposure. Kushelevsky (1949) reported on 25 patients who developed emphysema and bronchial asthma after blast exposures in World War II, but the cause of injury was not solely blast but dust and inhalation. That case series is reminiscent of possible health effects in people who were near the World Trade Center collapse in 2001; the effects of exposure to the dust generated in the collapse have been studied but have not been followed up in the context of blast exposure (Aldrich et al., 2010). Leone et al. (2008) reported on long-term outcomes in 91 survivors of multiple trauma with chest trauma and pulmonary contusions. Followup after 6 months and 1 year showed reduced measures of lung function, but the mechanism of injury was not blast exposure (in 80%, it was motor vehicle collisions), and the study was unable to differentiate between outcomes of chest trauma and outcomes of other injuries. Finally, Svennevig et al. (1989) looked at long-term outcomes in 24 patients who had closed-chest injuries and were treated a mean of 4.9 years (range 2–9 years) previously; there was no clear documentation of inclusion criteria or mechanism of case-series selection, and the mechanism of injury was not discussed, so the results that showed 63% with some pulmonary complaint at followup are not very useful for the present review.

There is a further literature, not specific to blast, that suggests that respiratory complaints in general, and the specific pathologic diagnosis of constrictive bronchiolitis in particular, are more common among those who have returned from Iraq and Afghanistan (Coker et al., 1999; King et al., 2011; Smith et al., 2009). Further, blast might be an important mediator of dust exposure. For example, a common, significant, and persistent decline in pulmonary function has been found to be associated with dust exposure in firefighters at the World Trade Center site (Aldrich et al., 2010). However, the literature review did not find compelling studies examining a specific role of blast in the development of these complaints, either directly or via dust exposure.

## Conclusions

Acute injuries to the respiratory tract are quite common after blasts. They range from burns in the upper airway to a classic syndrome of acute lung injury known as BLI. BLI is associated with high mortality and may require intensive care, including invasive mechanical ventilation. Blast exposure also can lead to serious acute whole-body inflammation (a risk factor for acute respiratory distress syndrome), and convalescent care for this puts patients at risk for the entire spectrum of PICS in the short and long term.

Despite the obvious acute injuries and the high plausibility of long-term sequelae, there is a striking absence of data on the long-term pulmonary outcomes of exposure to blast. That is true both of all who have been exposed to blast and of the subset of patients who develop acute BLI that requires care. Furthermore, the possibility of other long-term pulmonary consequences of blast exposure, such as the effect of explosion-related dust exposure, and of other exposures, such as smoking, has not been adequately examined.

The available studies are of insufficient quality, validity, consistency, or statistical power to support a conclusion regarding an association between exposure to blast and long-term respiratory outcomes in humans.

The committee concludes, on the basis of its evaluation, that there is inadequate/insufficient evidence of an association between exposure to blast and long-term effects on pulmonary function, respiratory symptoms, and exercise limitation.

The committee concludes, on the basis of its evaluation, that there is inadequate/insufficient evidence of long-term effects after acute blast lung injury.

## DIGESTIVE SYSTEM OUTCOMES

Primary blast injuries of the abdomen can cause severe damage to internal organs, typically in the absence of visible external signs of injury (Scekic et al., 1991). A recent review by Owers et al. (2011) examined the published literature on abdominal primary blast injury (PBI). According to the reviewed literature, the estimated overall incidence of abdominal PBI in hospitalized survivors of open-air blast explosions was about 3%; rates were marginally higher in those exposed to enclosed-space explosions. The incidence of abdominal PBI is generally much lower than that of PBI to the auditory and pulmonary systems (Owers et al., 2011); however, abdominal injuries may be more predominant in underwater blast explosions (Huller and Bazini, 1970). Laceration of solid organs (including abdominal organs) is rare and is associated with very high blast forces or proximity of the person to the explosion (DePalma et al., 2005) or with tertiary injury (Leibovici et al., 1996). More common, however, is PBI to gas-containing organs (Phillips and Richmond, 1991). Damage to those organs from PBI includes hemorrhage and perforations—particularly of the bowel—mesenteric shearing and hematoma, and ruptures of the hollow abdominal viscera (CDC, 2008a; Wani et al., 2009).

### Acute Effects

Signs and symptoms of blast injury to the abdomen can be readily apparent or nuanced and variable. Symptoms of gastrointestinal PBI include abdominal pain, nausea, testicular pain, tenesmus, and temporary loss of motor control in legs (CDC, 2008a; Phillips and Richmond, 1991). Signs of gastrointestinal PBI are similar to those of blunt trauma and may include abdominal and rebound tenderness, vomiting (hematemesis in rare occasions), voluntary and involuntary guarding, absence of or decrease in bowel sounds, rectal bleeding, and unexplained hypovolemia (Phillips and Richmond, 1991; Wani et al., 2009).

There is a degree of variability in the latency of the effects of PBI to the gastrointestinal tract, ranging from immediate onset to several years (Owers et al., 2011). A typical acute gastrointestinal mural hematoma can have delayed perforation up to 14 days after exposure (Owers et al., 2011). Late perforations usually occur within 2 weeks of the PBI (Scekic et al., 1991). Patients who have minor abdominal complaints may temporarily improve but then develop an abdominal crisis several weeks later (Phillips and Richmond, 1991).

## Long-Term Effects

To evaluate the long-term gastrointestinal health effects of blast exposure, the committee reviewed about 75 peer-reviewed studies. None met enough of the inclusion guidelines to be considered primary. This section details supportive studies of long-term gastrointestinal health outcomes of blast exposure.

The study that met the most inclusion guidelines was a retrospective chart review by Sayer et al. (2008) of patients admitted to four PRCs during 2001–2006. It evaluated a sample of 188 blast-exposed and non-blast-exposed veterans who sustained injuries in the Iraq and Afghanistan wars. Of the 188 patients, 56% had blast-related injuries. The measures used included scores on functional tests (functional independence measure within 72 hours of admission and at discharge) and length of stay. The study looked at a variety of health outcomes (not only gastrointestinal) and sought to quantify differences in outcomes between blast-exposed and non-blast-exposed patients. The results showed no significant difference in gastrointestinal injuries or gastrointestinal impairment between the two groups. However, the study has limitations for understanding possible long-term gastrointestinal effects in that the median length of stay (observed time frame) was only 29 days. In addition, the study did not look at specific gastrointestinal outcomes but instead aggregated all gastrointestinal injuries and impairments.

A study by Yzermans et al. (2005), reported on health outcomes of victims affected by a fireworks depot explosion in the Netherlands in which 22 people died immediately and more than 1,000 were injured. This retrospective longitudinal study aimed to quantify health problems (psychologic, medically unexplained, and gastrointestinal symptoms) and predictors of health problems. Electronic medical records from general practitioners' offices were examined to gather pre-disaster baseline morbidity (for the 16 months before the explosion) and post-disaster data for 2.5 years. The study was able to track 89% (9,329) of people exposed to the explosion and established a control group 7,392 matched for age and sex. The exposed group was also divided into two groups—those who had to relocate after the disaster and those who did not—to test the hypothesis that relocated disaster victims would have more health complaints than nonrelocated victims. The study showed a small increase in gastrointestinal morbidity in both groups compared with pre-disaster rates and control-group rates. Gastrointestinal complaints (for example, nausea and abdominal pain) were more prevalent in relocated victims after the disaster and throughout the whole period than in the control group. The study has several limitations for the purposes of the committee's charge to identify long-term health outcomes of blast exposure. First, the study did not gather data on exposure specific to the blast, so it is unclear what types of exposure and acute injuries the victims sustained and what mechanisms caused the injuries. Second, it reported general gastrointestinal complaints as an outcome, and this does not provide specific information about possible specific long-term gastrointestinal conditions that may result from the exposure. Third, although the study looked at socioeconomic status as a predictor of general gastrointestinal complaints, the controls were not matched for socioeconomic status.

A retrospective study by Ramasamy et al. (2012) met the guidelines only for a tertiary study but is worth mentioning because it provided long-term data on military personnel who were exposed to blast injuries. The study used a prospectively compiled combat-trauma registry of patients who sustained open pelvic blast injury during military service in Afghanistan. Of the 89 service personnel who had open pelvic fracture due to an explosion, 29 (33%) survived; 19 (66%) of the survivors had abdominal injuries. One-third of the patients had fecal diversion with a colostomy; all had either anal-sphincter disruption or severe bowel injury. The mean followup period was 20.3 months (range, 13.2–29.9). At final followup, seven patients had some continuing fecal incontinence.

## Conclusions

Blast can cause substantial injury to abdominal organs—including the gastrointestinal tract, liver, and spleen—both acutely and over the long term. There is a consensus that blast can cause hematomas and perforations of the gastrointestinal tract and lacerations of the liver and spleen. Delayed perforations can occur 1–14 days after blast injury; the most frequent period is 3–5 days. On the basis of the available literature, the committee determined that the long-term gastrointestinal effects of blast exposure have not been well studied. No studies met the committee's guidelines to be considered primary, and few studies provided any support in determining long-term gastrointestinal health outcomes. One of the two studies that the committee could identify as secondary found a small increase in gastrointestinal morbidity during the 2.5 years after blast exposure. However, the studies presented little detail on specific gastrointestinal injury and illness. Fecal incontinence is a long-term effect in people who have blast-associated severe bowel injury and anal-sphincter disruption. It is plausible that severe acute gastrointestinal injury can have long-term complications. For example, it is well known clinically that people who have had gastrointestinal surgery can develop bowel obstructions and that perforation of the intestine can have late complications that require an ileostomy or colostomy. In addition, it is possible that blast may cause dysfunction in the gastrointestinal system and brain–gut axis (the relationship between digestive health and mental health) that may go undetected in the immediate acute period or develop in the long term and become manifested in chronic symptoms, including abdominal pain and abnormal bowel habits.

The committee concludes, on the basis of its evaluation, that there is limited/suggestive evidence of an association between exposure to blast and acute gastrointestinal perforations and hemorrhages, and solid-organ laceration, all of which can have long-term consequences.

The committee concludes, on the basis of its evaluation, that there is inadequate/insufficient evidence of an association between exposure to blast in the absence of a serious acute injury and long-term gastrointestinal outcomes.

## GENITOURINARY OUTCOMES

Genitourinary (GU) injury includes injury to the upper urinary tract (kidneys and ureters), the lower urinary tract (bladder and urethra), and the external genitalia (penis, scrotum, and testicles). The literature on GU blast injuries almost exclusively describes injury to males. GU injury to female service members has not been well described in the literature and so was not a focus of this report.

### Acute Effects

The committee identified several recent studies of acute GU injury that resulted from blast exposure in combat in the Iraq and Afghanistan wars.

A retrospective review by Serkin et al. (2010) found that of the 16,323 US service member trauma admissions logged into the JTTR in October 2001–January 2008, 819 (5%) involved one or more GU injuries. Explosions or blast caused 65.3% of these injuries. The scrotum was the GU organ most commonly injured, and 82.8% of scrotal injuries were caused by explosion. A smaller review of GU trauma at a combat support hospital in Iraq from April 2005 through February 2006 looked at 2,712 admissions, and 76 (2.8%) were for GU injuries, 50% of which were caused by a blast or explosive ordinance (Paquette, 2007). A retrospective review by Fleming et al. (2012) looked at trauma patients treated at the National Naval Medical Center (NNMC) who had sustained injuries in the Iraq and Afghanistan wars during September 2007–December 2010. This review focused on patients who had major-extremity amputations and examined the number and type of associated injuries. Most of the patients included in the study had blast injuries from IEDs; the injuries of 62 of the 63 patients who had multiple extremity amputations and of 37 of the 46 who had single extremity amputations were caused by blast. The authors found that multiple extremity amputations correlated with GU injuries, which included injuries to the external genitalia, the bladder, and the urethra. The 63 patients who had multiple extremity amputations had a total of 71 GU injuries (specific types of injuries were not stated, and several patients had multiple GU injuries), whereas the 46 patients who had single extremity amputations had 29 GU injuries (specific types of injuries were not stated). Another recent paper examined the UK JTTR for the Iraq and Afghanistan wars from 2003 to 2010. Of the 2,204 registered patients, 85 (3.9%) had GU injuries; the percentage who sustained GU injuries from blast was not stated (Mossadegh et al., 2012).

Andersen et al. (2012) noted that since additional troops were deployed to Afghanistan in 2010, there has been an increase in the incidence of GU trauma in US service members. The increase presumably is due in part to the nature of combat operations in Afghanistan, where terrain necessitates more patrolling on foot by dismounted troops, who are at particular risk for being injured by blast explosions from IEDs without the protection of an armored vehicle. The authors also discuss the effects of better surgical and trauma care on the battlefield, which has resulted in a greater number of survivors who have complex blast injuries, including multiple-extremity amputation patients. In prior wars, casualties with such extensive injuries more frequently failed to survive to evacuation out of theater.

A similar article by Mossadegh et al. (2012) that looked at the British experience with troops deployed to Afghanistan and Iraq from 2003 to 2010 comments on blast injuries in these conflicts as more likely to cause higher, transfemoral amputations than in other conflicts (for example, Bosnia-Herzogovena), in which explosive devices were more likely to be land mines and more likely to cause below-knee amputations. IED blasts were also more likely to cause perineal injuries and pelvic fractures. Of the 2,204 patients registered in the UK JTTR, 118 had perineal injuries, and 85 of these patients (72%) had GU injuries. Of the 118 patients who had perineal injuries, 56 (47%) eventually died of their wounds. The combination of a perineal wound and a pelvic fracture resulted in the highest mortality (73%) in these 118 patients. A pelvic fracture alone was associated with mortality of 41% and a perineal injury with mortality of 18%. Eight of the 85 patients who had GU injuries had complete testicular loss.

### Long-Term Effects

The committee reviewed about 40 peer-reviewed studies of GU health effects of blast exposure. None of the studies met the committee's inclusion guidelines for primary studies; supportive studies are discussed below. However, the committee determined that there are expected long-term GU effects on the basis of the nature of acute injuries that have been documented. As discussed above, recent studies of combat-trauma casualties have shown that acute GU injuries are commonly caused by blast exposures such as those from IEDs (Andersen et al., 2012; Fleming et al., 2012; Mossadegh et al., 2012; Paquette, 2007; Serkin et al., 2010). Expected long-term health outcomes related to the types of acute GU injuries caused by blast exposure would be hypogonadism, infertility, erectile dysfunction, and voiding dysfunction. The committee determined that although these long-term health outcomes have not been studied in relation specifically to blast exposure, it is logical to assume that they could result from the acute GU injuries commonly incurred from exposure to blast.

The hypogonadism is caused by direct loss of testicular tissue because of a blast injury to the scrotum in addition to posttraumatic hypopituitarism from mild TBI caused by a blast injury. The anterior pituitary seems to be particularly sensitive to blast injury: there is a secondary decrease in release of follicle-stimulating hormone (FSH) and luteinizing hormone (LH) and a consequent decrease in release of testosterone from the testicles. Wilkinson et al. (2012) examined 26 service members who had mild TBI caused by a blast and compared them with a control group of 59 veterans who had similar deployment history but no history of blast injury or head trauma and normal cognitive testing. Eleven (42%) of the 26 in the mild-TBI group had some abnormality in hormones from the anterior pituitary; none in the control group had any such abnormalities. Three patients had hypogonadism as shown by serum testosterone concentrations in less than the 5th percentile of normal reference ranges, coupled with FSH and LH concentrations in less than the 10th percentile of normal reference ranges.

Low testosterone decreases sex drive and muscle mass and leads to anemia, osteoporosis, low energy, and possibly depression.

Wilkinson et al. (2012) also demonstrated a growth hormone deficiency (GHD) that occurred in five of the 26 veterans in the mild-TBI blast group and none of the control group. Growth hormone concentrations were measured indirectly on the basis of insulin-like growth factor-1 (IGF-1) concentrations; IGF-1 concentrations less than the 10th percentile of reference concentrations are thought to represent GHD. GHD decreases sex drive, strength, muscle volume, and metabolic rate. Wilkinson et al. (2012) demonstrated that those changes persist for up to 1 year. The remaining patients in the study who had hormone abnormalities had low oxytocin concentrations: two veterans had increased vasopressin concentrations (over the 95th percentile) and two had decreased vasopressin concentrations (under the 5th percentile).

Baxter et al. (2013) conducted complete endocrine evaluations of 19 UK service members for 2–48 months after they received moderate to severe blast TBI (as discussed above, neuroimaging and cognitive assessment also were conducted). They compared that group with 39 control patients. In the control non-blast-TBI group, injuries were secondary to motor vehicle collisions (43%), assaults (32%), falls (23%), and sporting injuries (2%). Six of 19 (32%) service members who had blast TBI but only 1 of 39 (2.6%) controls had anterior pituitary dysfunction (p = 0.004). Two service members who had blast TBI had hyperprolactinemia, two had GHD, one had adrenocorticotropic hormone deficiency, and one had combined GHD, adrenocorticotropic hormone deficiency, and gonadotropin deficiency. Four of the 19 patients in the blast-TBI group had hypogonadism secondary to direct blast injury to the testicles and perineum; these 4 had normal anterior pituitary function. The five patients in the blast-TBI group who had hypogonadism are examples of how direct blast injury and hypopituitarism as a result of blast affect testosterone production; all five will need lifelong testosterone replacement therapy.

Loss of testicular tissue can also result in infertility in this population of young men. The effects of low FSH and LH in the Wilkinson et al. (2012) and Baxter et al. (2013) studies discussed above also could result in infertility (sperm production depends on both hormones but primarily on FSH); however, this effect was not examined in those studies or other studies reviewed by the committee.

Direct injury to the penis from a blast can result in erectile dysfunction (ED), which can have important long-term emotional effects in this young population. The ED is caused by damage of the corporal bodies or erectile nerves to the penis and interruption of blood flow to and from the penis, which results from substantial pelvic trauma. Complex phallic reconstruction techniques are feasible in patients who have suffered blast injury to the penis (Peker et al., 2002). Long-term studies looking at ED in patients who suffered blast injuries have not been performed.

Voiding dysfunction in patients after blast injury has not been well described, but several studies have looked at voiding dysfunction in patients who have sustained a TBI from events other than a military blast injury (usually motor vehicle collisions). The studies found a wide variation of abnormalities, from hyperactive bladder to hypoactive bladder, depending on the nature and location of and time since neurologic injury (Ersoz et al., 2011; Giannantoni et al., 2011).

Bladder and urethral injuries after a blast injury often require a series of complex reconstructive surgeries and can lead to urethral strictures and incontinence. Long-term outcomes of patients who have had urethral reconstruction after blast injuries have not been adequately described.

More than 643,000 US veterans of the Iraq and Afghanistan wars were examined to assess the association between lower urinary tract symptoms (LUTS) and PTSD. *International Classification of Diseases, Ninth Revision* (ICD-9) codes were used to identify LUTS and PTSD. Male veterans who had PTSD were more likely to have LUTS than those who did not have PTSD (2.9% vs 1.1%; p < 0.001) (Breyer et al., 2012). The same database was used to examine the association between PTSD and sexual dysfunction (ED and premature ejaculation). Male veterans who had PTSD were more likely than those who do not have PTSD to suffer from sexual dysfunction (9.8% vs 3.3%; p < 0.001) (Breyer et al., 2012).

## Conclusions

On the basis of expert clinical knowledge, the committee knows that exposure to blast can lead acutely to complete functional and structural loss of GU organs. The committee found two studies that reported on long-term GU health outcomes of blast exposure (Baxter et al., 2013; Wilkinson et al., 2012). The studies showed persistent hypogonadism as a result of hypopituitarism in some patients up to 2 years after TBI from a blast. For example, if a soldier has an acute blast injury and loss of both testicles and trauma to the penis that results in damage to the corporal bodies and urethra, he will have permanent, long-term problems with hypogonadism, infertility, voiding dysfunction, and ED. The answer to the clinical question, How much does a partial injury to a GU organ contribute to long-term consequences from blast injuries?, is unknown because studies are lacking.

**The committee concludes, on the basis of its evaluation, that there is sufficient evidence of a causal relationship between exposure to blast and some long-term effects on a genitourinary organ—such as hypogonadism, infertility, voiding dysfunction, and erectile dysfunc-**

tion—associated with severe injury (defined as a complete structural and functional loss that cannot be reconstructed).

The committee concludes, on the basis of its evaluation, that there is inadequate/insufficient evidence of an association between exposure to blast and long-term effects associated with partial injury to a genitourinary organ (defined as an incomplete structural and functional loss that can be reconstructed).

## DERMAL OUTCOMES

Information on dermal outcomes other than direct outcomes of burns from exposure to blast is sparse. Mesquita-Guimaraes et al. (1987) reported on a patient who presented with multiple silica granulomas on the left side of his body. Fifteen years earlier, while in military service, he had stepped on a land mine that exploded, and that led to amputation of his left leg and numerous other injuries. His injuries healed, but numerous black particles remained embedded in his skin. Three years after the explosion, the patient had inflammation around the particles in his left forearm; the condition resolved with unspecified topical medication and antibiotics. X-ray spectroscopy of the particles showed them to be silica, possibly from the earth that was disrupted by the land mine. The authors believe that over the years the silica slowly converted to colloidal silica, which can cause nonallergic foreign-body reactions. In another case report, Wijekoon et al. (1995) reported a case in a 29-year-old man of sarcoid-like granulomatous skin lesions at sites that were exposed to a bomb blast 7 years earlier. The authors hypothesized that the granulomas were produced by foreign material that was embedded in the skin during the blast. In a third case report, a 14-year-old girl developed prurigo nodularis–like skin eruptions about 4 months after a bomb blast (Ghosh et al., 2009). The lesions were in the same place (her arms and face) as the original blast injury and initially consisted of multiple tiny burn injuries. The skin condition improved markedly with topical glucocorticoid and hydroxyzine use. No long-term cohort studies have reported on dermal sequelae of blast injuries not directly related to burns. However, although few studies were found, the committee concludes on the basis of expert clinical knowledge that exposure to blast can have dermal effects.

The committee concludes, on the basis of its evaluation, that there is sufficient evidence of an association between exposure to blast and long-term dermal effects, such as cutaneous granulomas.

## MUSCULOSKELETAL AND REHABILITATION OUTCOMES

The musculoskeletal system and soft-tissue areas have the highest incidence of bodily injuries in blast survivors, the most extreme being traumatic amputation, which occurs in 1–3% of blast victims (CDC, 2008b). Those injuries can be manifested as primary, secondary, tertiary, or quaternary; any of them can occur alone or in combination (Covey, 2002). Musculoskeletal primary blast injuries caused by the blast wave or wind usually occur in proximity to the explosion and result primarily in traumatic amputation. That is a fairly rare outcome because of the high associated mortality, but there has been an increase in traumatic-amputation survivors owing to advances in medicine and body-armor technology (Covey, 2002; Mody et al., 2009). Secondary blast injury predominates as the most common blast injury to the musculoskeletal system and is most often the result of penetration by shrapnel and other fragments, which causes trauma ranging from minor lacerations to deep embedding of foreign bodies. Nonpenetrating contusions and bone fractures are also possible (CDC, 2008b). Tertiary and quaternary blast injuries to the musculoskeletal system are rare and mostly follow a pattern similar to that of civilian trauma from blunt-impact forces. Contusions, lacerations, and fractures are all possible, and crush injuries may result in compartment syndrome (CDC, 2008b). As of December 2012, the total number of amputations (of major limbs, such as a leg, and minor limbs, such as s finger) in military personnel serving in Iraq and Afghanistan was 1,715 (Fischer, 2013).

### Acute Effects

Injuries to the musculoskeletal system are generally overt and easy to diagnose on the basis of outward signs and victim-reported symptoms; however, a few complications can arise and should be suspected with blast injuries. In many cases, soft-tissue injury extends well beyond the zone of skin and bone damage (CDC, 2008b). One of the biggest concerns in connection with blast injuries to the musculoskeletal system is wound contamination and the high risk of complicated and potentially lethal infection (CDC, 2008b; Covey, 2002). Of particular concern with regard to infection are open bone fractures (especially of long bones) and traumatic implantation of shrapnel, dirt, and biologic material, including bone fragments from other victims (Mody et al., 2009). Blast injuries contaminated with *Aeromonas hydrophilia*, an organism not commonly found in civilian musculoskeletal injuries, are associated with the requirement for a more proximal amputation (Penn-Barwell et al., 2012). Additional information about infections related to exposure to blast appears later in this chapter. Finally, because of the pattern of polytrauma in blast injuries, musculoskeletal injuries are often markers of damage to other organ systems, such as cardiovascular and neurologic damage in extremities (CDC, 2008b).

## Long-Term Effects

To evaluate the long-term musculoskeletal and rehabilitation outcomes of blast exposure, the committee reviewed about 70 peer-reviewed studies. None of the studies met enough of the inclusion guidelines to be considered primary. This section details supportive studies on musculoskeletal and rehabilitation outcomes of blast exposure.

Sayer et al. (2008) is particularly informative in that it separated blast-injured and non-blast-injured patients to compare their outcomes (the study examined cognitive and motor functional gain scores and length of stay). The results showed no significant difference between blast and non-blast patients in orthopedic, fracture, amputation, and pain outcomes. In blast patients, several types of injuries were found to be more common: oral and maxillofacial ($p < 0.05$) and skin or soft-tissue injury ($p < 0.001$), including burns ($p < 0.05$) and wounds ($p < 0.001$). The study is generally informative with respect to the functional status of blast versus non-blast patients during the rehabilitation period after injury, but it has limitations in providing evidence on specific long-term musculoskeletal and rehabilitation outcomes of blast. The study did not include an objective measure of blast exposure at the time of injury and instead identified blast exposure on the basis of self-reporting in the medical chart. In addition, as mentioned previously in the review of gastrointestinal outcomes, the study has limitations for understanding possible long-term effects in that the median period of observation of patients' functioning was just 29 days. Although the blast and non-blast groups were found not to be different at discharge in functional gain after rehabilitation, the study does not indicate whether there were long-term differences between the two groups.

Using US Army Physical Evaluation Board medical records, Rivera et al. (2012) assessed the prevalence of osteoarthritis in 1,566 combat-injured US service members who could not return to duty. Of the 1,566, 126 cases of osteoarthritis were identified. Sites of osteoarthritis were knee, elbow, ankle, shoulder, foot, wrist, spine, and hip. Eighty-one percent of the service members were exposed to blast. Only 10% of the 126 service members had osteoarthritis before deployment. A case report also describes the development of osteoarthritis in a service member who was exposed to blast (Coy and Chatfield, 1998). The soldier was exposed to blast and sustained multiple injuries, including bilateral soft-tissue shrapnel injuries to his legs and hyperextension of his knees, while serving in the Vietnam War. He developed knee pain and arthritis within 10 years of sustaining the initial injuries.

Several other studies provided information on long-term musculoskel-etal and rehabilitation outcomes. The development of heterotopic ossifica-tion (the presence of bone in soft tissue where bone does not normally exist) has been reported in a residual limb in up to 63% of combat-related amputations (Potter et al., 2007); this finding is unexpected because hetero-topic ossification was a rare complication of amputation before the conflicts in Iraq and Afghanistan (Alfieri et al., 2012). Forsberg et al. (2009), in a retrospective cohort study, aimed to understand the prevalence and risk factors for heterotopic ossification in combat-wounded patients who were admitted to NNMC from March 1, 2003, through December 31, 2006. The study group consisted of 157 patients who had undergone at least one orthopedic procedure on an extremity and developed heterotopic ossifica-tion; 86 patients who did not develop heterotopic ossification made up the control group. Followup of patients included in the study ranged from 2–41 months (mean, 8.4 months) for the heterotopic ossification group and from 2–36 months (mean, 7.1 months) for the control group. Mechanism of injury was specifically examined to determine whether heterotopic ossi-fication was associated with one injury type rather than another. Results of the record review showed a relationship between blast injury and devel-opment of heterotopic ossification, but the relationship only approached significance (p = 0.06). In a univariate analysis, however, blast injury with concurrent TBI or an injury severity score (ISS) of at least 16 was predictive of heterotopic ossification (p = 0.02 and 0.04, respectively).

Dougherty (1999) carried out a record review to identify bilateral above-knee amputation patients treated at Valley Forge General Hospital during the Vietnam War and then conducted followup interviews to report on their long-term outcomes. Of the 30 identified patients, 26 (87%) had been injured by land mines or booby traps. At followup (an average of 27.5 years after the injury), the 23 patients who responded were found to have lower physical function (statistically significant with p < 0.01) than matched controls on the 36-question short-form health survey. There were no differences between groups in physical-role functioning, bodily pain, general health, vitality, social functioning, and mental health functioning. The study did not separate blast-injured and non-blast-injured patients, so any reported differences in functional status between the groups cannot be attributed specifically to blast.

A retrospective review by Cross et al. (2012) reported on 115 Army service members who sustained battle-related open tibia fractures. The study examined whether the service members returned to duty and, if they were unable to return, what disability rating they acquired. Results showed an overall return-to-duty rate of 18% among the service members and a 12.5% rate in those who had amputations. The mechanism of injury of 78% of the service members was explosion (88% of the amputees sustained injuries that were due to explosion). Although the study indicates that amputation and medical retirement are frequent in those who have open tibia fractures caused by blast, it did not compare the long-term health outcomes between those who were blast-exposed and those who were non-blast-exposed. The study also has limitations in its usefulness for the committee's review owing to its small sample and its use of return to duty as the main outcome examined.

A retrospective review by Tintle et al. (2012) reported on 96 patients, all US military personnel, who suffered 100 upper-extremity amputations during October 2004–April 2009. The study examined outcomes and operative complications, types of complications, and frequency of revision surgery after upper-extremity amputations as a result of combat-related trauma. Of the amputations, 87% resulted from exposure to blast and an additional 8% were due to high-velocity gunshot wounds. Nearly half the amputations—42%—were followed by at least one complication that required revision. Deep infection led to 51% of the revision procedures. Heterotopic ossification was another cause of revision procedures: It occurred in 66% of the 63 limbs that had at least 2 months of radiographic followup (not all patients had radiographic followup). Other complications were neuromas (excised in 9% of the limbs), wound dehiscence (6%), need for scar revision (5%), and need for contracture release (4%). The records indicate that all the patients had a completely healed residual limb at final followup. Continuing phantom-limb pain and residual-limb pain were reported in 37% and 51% of the patients, respectively. Pain status was not recorded for all patients.

Feldt et al. (2013) conducted a retrospective review by using data from the Joint Facial and Invasive Neck Trauma Project to assess the numbers and types of facial and penetrating neck injuries sustained by US military personnel serving in Iraq and Afghanistan from January 2003 through May 2011. The number of discrete facial and penetrating neck injuries identified was 37,523; they occurred in 7,177 service members. Exposure to blast was the mechanism of injury in 24.2% of the cases. Other mechanisms were penetrating trauma (49.1%), blunt trauma (25.7%), and other or unknown or burns (1%). The study did not report on long-term outcomes.

Another study of US military personnel serving in Iraq and Afghanistan assessed facial injuries, specifically mandibular fractures, by using JTTR data (Zachar et al., 2013). Data from October 2001 to April 2011 were analyzed, and 391 patients who had mandibular fractures were identified. The mechanisms of injury in those patients were exposure to blast (61.3%), ballistics (12.5%), and motor vehicle collisions (1%). The fracture patterns in the service members differed somewhat from those in the general population, possibly because of the mechanisms of injury: service members were exposed more to blast, whereas mechanisms of injury in civilians are typically motor vehicle collisions, interpersonal violence, and falls. The study also did not report on long-term outcomes.

A third study consisted of a retrospective review of US service members who sustained facial injuries during the Iraq war and were treated from April to October 2006 (Salinas and Faulkner, 2010). The 21 patients were identified by one of the study authors, who treated the injured service members in Iraq. The study compared outcomes in patients who were treated immediately in theater and outcomes in patients whose treatment was delayed until after transport out of theater. Overall, the mechanism of injury was exposure to blast in 57% of the patients—in 43% of the immediately treated group and 86% in the delayed-treatment group. Treatment of blast-exposed patients may have been more often delayed because their injuries were more severe and required more complex procedures that were available only in facilities that were out of theater. The complication rate was 24% (five complications in four patients). Four of the complications were infections. A limitation of the study is the small population (21 patients).

Koc et al. (2008) reported on long-term skin problems in 142 amputees in Turkey. The time between initial amputation and enrollment in the study ranged from 1 to 21 years. The results showed that amputees had a high prevalence of skin problems (73.9%), and the study also reported differences between those using soft pocket prostheses and those using silicone prostheses. Although the study documented that 80.3% of the amputations were caused by mine explosions, there was no comparison of those who suffered blast injuries with those who did not. Therefore, the study is not useful in understanding whether long-term skin problems in amputees can be attributed specifically to blast injury. Additional information about dermal effects is presented in the preceding section of this chapter.

## Conclusion

Exposure to blast has several obvious outcomes, such as loss of limbs and scarring. Few studies of other outcomes related to blast exposure and the musculoskeletal system and rehabilitation were identified. There is some evidence that blast-related amputations result in a higher incidence of complications, including heterotopic ossification in those requiring amputations, and osteoarthritis.

**The committee concludes, on the basis of its evaluation, that there is limited/suggestive evidence of an association between exposure to blast and long-term consequences for the musculoskeletal system, including heterotopic ossification in amputee limbs and osteoarthritis.**

## INFECTIONS

Infections in blast-exposed people can be caused directly by blast and can be acquired indirectly during administration of medical care after exposure to a blast. With respect to most of the studies on complications from infections described below, it was not possible for the committee to determine whether an infectious organism was introduced into a wound (during a blast or during later medical care).

Infection remains a common problem for veterans. Of 2.2 million Iraq and Afghanistan war veterans, 144,167 (0.07%) have been treated for problems related to infectious diseases (ICD-9 codes 001–139) in VA medical facilities since 2001 (VA, 2013). Pathogenic bacteria are commonly found in the wounds of military personnel who have blast injuries (Murray, 2008a,b). An infection rate of 5.5% was reported in an assessment of JTTR data on infection-related complications in combat casualties in the Iraq and Afghanistan wars (Murray et al., 2011). A retrospective chart review published in 2009 provides a summary of infections identified in Iraq and Afghanistan veterans treated in a PRC in the Palo Alto Health Care System (Dau et al., 2009). The authors reviewed patient records from the period January 2002–October 2007. During that time, 180 veterans received care in the unit, and 35 (19%) developed 137 unique infections while in the hospital. The most common isolates were from the urinary tract (26%), followed by sputum (23%), wound (18%), and blood (15%); bacteria of 21 species were recovered (see Table 4-4). Many of the veterans had polymicrobial infections, and many of the infections were trauma-related (that is, the wounds were caused by or related to high-velocity projectiles, blast devices, and burns). Gram-positive microorganisms and anaerobes predominated at the time of injury, but gram-negative organisms caused later infections in the wounds.

Fungi also have been isolated from the wounds of military personnel who served in Iraq and Afghanistan (Paolino et al., 2012; Warkentien et al., 2012). Organisms include the genera *Absidia, Biopolaris, Fusarium*, and *Mucor* and several species of *Aspergillus*. Nearly all the military personnel in those studies received their wounds from exposure to blast. Candidemia has been reported in people who have been exposed to blast (Wolf et al., 2000).

Infected wounds are commonly caused by explosives, such as IEDs (Murray, 2008a). The risk of infection from explosive devices can be increased by introduction of ground material and other matter added to the devices into the wounds. Injuries to the extremities are the most prevalent, followed by injuries to the head and neck, thorax, and abdomen. Burn-related infections complicate treatment of combat casualties. Burn patients are particularly susceptible to bacterial infections because of skin

**TABLE 4-4** Top Five Isolated Organisms by Site Cultured

| Culture Site (Total No. Isolates, % Total Infections) | Organism (No. Isolates[a]) |
|---|---|
| Blood (21, 15) | |
| 1 | Coagulase-negative *Staphylococcus* (14) |
| 2 | *Candida* sp. (2) |
| 3 | *Pseudomonas aeruginosa* (2) |
| 4–6 | *Enterobacter aerogenes, Enterococcus* sp., *Klebsiella pneumoniae* (ESBL) (1 each) |
| Sputum (31, 23) | |
| 1 | Methicillin-sensitive *Staphylococcus aureus* (6) |
| 2 | *Pseudomonas aeruginosa* (6) |
| 3 | *Klebsiella pneumoniae* (4, 2 ESBL) |
| 4 | *Stenotrophomonas maltophilia* (4) |
| 5 | *Acinetobacter baumannii* (3) |
| Urine[b] (36, 26) | |
| 1 | *Pseudomonas aeruginosa* (9) |
| 2 | *Klebsiella pneumoniae* (7, 3 ESBL) |
| 3 | *Escherichia coli* (6, 3 ESBL) |
| 4 | Methicillin-resistant *Staphylococcus aureus* (3) |
| 5 | *Enterobacter cloacae* (2) |
| Wound (25, 18) | |
| 1 | Methicillin-resistant *Staphylococcus aureus* (8) |
| 2 | Coagulase-negative *Staphylococcus* (4) |
| 3 | Methicillin-sensitive *Staphylococcus aureus* (4) |
| 4 | *Pseudomonas aeruginosa* (4) |
| 5 | *Acinetobacter baumannii, Enterobacter cloacae, Proteus mirabilis, Rhodotorula mucilaginosa, Streptococcus salivarius* (1 each) |
| Other (24, 18) | |
| 1 | *Pseudomonas aeruginosa* (5) |
| 2 | Coagulase-negative *Staphylococcus* (3) |
| 3 | *Clostridium difficile* (3) |
| 4 | *Enterococcus* sp. (3) |
| 5 | Methicillin-resistant *Staphylococcus aureus* (2) |

NOTE: ESBL = extended-spectrum-β-lactamase; sp = species.
[a]Top five organisms only; therefore, number may not match total number in left column.
[b]One urine culture was positive for *Acinetobacter*.
SOURCE: Dau et al., 2009.

breakdown and the risk of nosocomial infection in the hospital environment (Dau et al., 2009). Numerous studies in military and civilian populations have reported that infection with pathogens increases the risk of death and otherwise can complicate healing in burn patients, for example, Bennett et al. (2010), Calvano et al. (2010), D'Avignon et al. (2010), Horvath et al. (2007), Murray et al. (2008), Ressner et al. (2008), and

Schofield et al. (2007). Wounded personnel can be particularly susceptible to infection because of comorbid health problems (for example, immuno-suppression or subclinical conditions, such as sexually transmitted diseases or leishmaniasis).

During the Iraq and Afghanistan wars, multidrug-resistant (MDR) bacteria have been increasingly common (Dau et al., 2009; Keen et al., 2010; Murray, 2008a; Murray et al., 2009; Sherwood et al., 2011). There have been increases in casualties' MDR infections with such organisms as *Acinetobacter baumannii–calcoaceticus* complex, *Pseudomonas aeruginosa*, and *Klebsiella pneumoniae*.

The committee did not identify any studies that met its guidelines for primary studies, but did identify a number of supportive studies: a cohort study that is still going on, a case-control study, five retrospective chart reviews, and several case reports that provide information on acute and chronic complications from infections of wounds caused by blast.

## Acute Effects

Wolf et al. (2000) conducted a case control study of candidemia in people who were injured by a blast while visiting an outdoor food marketplace in Israel. The cases consisted of 21 patients injured in the marketplace. To be included in the study, the cases had to be hospitalized for more than 24 hours. Two control groups were used: The first consisted of 29 patients who had similar blast injuries from a different explosion at an open-air pedestrian mall (referred to as the blast-injury controls), and the second consisted of 40 ICU patients (referred to as the ICU controls) treated at the same time as the case patients. Within 4 days after injury, four of the cases had respiratory infections from *Aspergillus* or *Rhizopus*. Between 4 and 16 days, 7 of them developed candidemia (the *Candida* was not isolated from the wounds before being isolated from blood). Mortality in infected cases was 43%. Quantitative air sampling was conducted, and higher concentrations of *Aspergillus* and *Rhizopus* were found in the marketplace than in the pedestrian mall and *Candida* was found only in the marketplace. The incidence of *Candida* was significantly lower in the control groups than in the case group (p = 0.001 for the ICU controls and p = 0.02 for the blast-injury controls). The cluster of cases and the early temporal pattern suggest that infection occurred at the time of the blast rather than being hospital acquired, although nosocomial infection cannot be ruled out.

Albrecht et al. (2006) assessed medical records and microbiology-laboratory data of patients admitted to a US military tertiary-care burn center from January 2003 to November 2005. *Acinetobacter baumannii–calcoaceticus* complex infection was found in 59 of 802 burn patients. Mortality was higher in the infected patients; however, on multivariate analysis, infection did not independently affect mortality (p = 0.651). That result suggests that "although *Acinetobacter* is a marker of increased crude mortality because of its association with larger burns, it does not affect mortality independently" (Albrecht et al., 2006, p. 549). The authors did not report how many of the patients were military versus civilian (this burn center also receives civilian burn patients) or how many patients sustained their burns as a result of exposure to explosions.

Johnson et al. (2007a) reviewed infections in type III fractures (high-energy injuries typically with bone comminution or loss and lacerations of greater than 10 cm). Historically, type III fractures have a reported infection rate of 6–39% and an amputation rate of less than 10%. Thirty-five service members with type III open diaphyseal tibial fractures admitted to Brooks Army Medical Center (BAMC) during March 2003–August 2006 were identified through medical records. The mechanism of injury was an explosive device in 27 (77%) of the 35 cases. All patients had received irrigation and debridement before arriving at BAMC. During each patient's first surgical debridement at BAMC, samples for initial cultures were taken from deep tissues. Samples were taken again later. Before arriving at BAMC, all patients received perioperative antibiotics for gram positive bacteria. The mean evacuation time from injury to arrival at BAMC was 7.4 days. Of the 35 patients, 27 had infections at admission; the most common organisms were *Acinetobacter baumannii–calcoaceticus* complex, *Enterobacter* species, and *Pseudomonas aeruginosa*. All 27 received antibiotics; 24 (89%) received therapy for osteomyelitis, and the remaining three for deep-wound infection. Delayed union was another complication. Thirteen patients had deep-wound infections at reassessment, most of which were staphylococcal. Five of the 35 patients ultimately required amputation, and infection was the cause in 4 of the 5 cases. A limitation of this study is the small number of patients.

The goal of Paolino et al. (2012) was to determine the incidence of invasive fungal infections at WRAMC. They reviewed electronic medical records of military personnel sent to WRAMC from March 2002 to July 2008 with suspected invasive fungal infection and found six cases (three proved and three probable). All cases had been deployed to Iraq, and five had acquired blast injuries. The fungi in the cases were *Absidia*, several species of *Aspergillus*, *Biopolaris*, *Fusarium*, and *Mucor*. Three of the five cases required amputation of extremities or substantial revision of previous amputation sites. No deaths were noted.

Warkentien et al. (2012) used JTTR data to study fungal wound infections in military personnel who had extremity injuries due to blast. All patients were injured in Afghanistan and admitted to WRAMC, NNMC, or BAMC via Landstuhl Regional Medical Center in Germany from June 1, 2009, to December 31, 2010. Thirty-seven patients had diagnoses of fungal wound infections (20 proved, 4 probable, and 13 possible). The fungi found were *Aspergillus, Fusarium,* and *Mucorales.* Of the 37 patients, 33 received antifungal therapy. Twelve patients had amputations, but it is not clear whether the amputations were due specifically to the fungal infections. Five patients who had fungal infections died, and it was noted that the infections played a role in three of the deaths.

Silla et al. (2006) prospectively reviewed clinical records of 22 patients who were injured in a bombing in Bali on October 12, 2002. The patients were admitted to a burn unit in a hospital in Western Australia, and their records were compared with those of 37 burn patients in the same hospital who were not injured by blast. The incidence of primary burn-wound infection was statistically significantly higher in the Bali bombing patients (15 patients, 68%) than in the other burn patients (7 patients, 19%) (p = 0.001). Pathogens isolated from the Bali burn patients were *Pseudomonas aeruginosa, Staphylococcus aureus, Bacillus cereus, Enterococcus* species, MDR *Acinetobacter baumannii, Chryseobacterium indologenes, Candida, Enterobacter cloacae,* and *Diphtheroid bacillus*; the other patients were infected with *Pseudomonas aeruginosa, Klebsiella pneumoniae, Serrata marcescens,* and *Bacillus cereus.* All Bali bombing patients received antibiotic prophylaxis before arriving at the burn unit, whereas only 5 of the 37 other patients received it. The patients were not followed for a long period.

*Pseudomonas putida* was identified in a member of the US military who sustained injuries in an explosion in Iraq (Carpenter et al., 2008). Bilateral transtibial amputations were performed on the day of the explosion and the patient was ultimately transferred to NNMC, where after 10 days he developed leukocytosis, high fever, and purulent drainage from the right leg stump. *Pseudomonas putida* was cultured from the wound site, and the patient was treated with intravenous meropenem for 14 days; there were no further infectious complications.

## Long-Term Effects

Tribble et al. (2011) published a preliminary report on a continuing cohort study with an observational design that is assessing short- and long-term outcomes of infections after deployment-related traumatic injury. Participants are enrolled while hospitalized at WRAMC, BAMC, or NNMC. They will be followed for 5 years via interviews, Web-based questionnaires, and review of DOD and VA electronic medical records. Patient trauma and surgical history is obtained by using JTTR data. Of 354 patients, 180 (52%) were exposed to blast, and 69 patients (31.7% of those exposed) had an infection. At 6-month followup after discharge, there were 28 incident infections (bloodstream infections, skin and soft-tissue infections, osteomyelitis, pneumonia, sinusitis, urinary tract infection, and *Clostridium difficile* infection). In about 15% of cases, continuing management for the infections was needed. The study is continuing to enroll participants.

Brown et al. (2010) conducted a retrospective chart review to study infections in British service members who had sustained life-threatening and limb-threatening injuries in the Iraq and Afghanistan wars. They had undergone limb-salvage procedures for severely mangled extremity injuries, all of which resulted from blast or ballistics. The authors used JTTR data from August 12, 2003 through August 2007 (the last followup was in May 2008) to review trauma audit and clinical records. Eighty-four casualties with 85 extremity injuries were available for analysis, and 20 of the casualties had infections. The more severely injured had higher infection rates, and there were more infections in wounds of the lower extremities than of the upper extremities. No differences were found between infected and noninfected patients in ISS, time from injury to evacuation, time from injury to surgery, or time to arrival in England. More infectious complications were associated with injuries that required fasciotomy; no association was found between infectious complications and use of hemorrhage control in the field (for example, QuickClot and HemCon dressings). Bacteria initially recovered included *Acinetobacter* species, *Pseudomonas aeruginosa*, and *Staphylococcus aureus*. Other bacteria recovered later during the course of recovery were *Aeromonas* species, *Bacillus* species, *Chryseobacterium* species, *Clostridium* species, *Enterobacter* species, *Escherichia coli*, *Klebsiella* species, methicillin-resistant *Staphylococcus aureus*, and *Stenotrophomonas* species. Two of the patients' extremities had recovery of *Pseudomonas aeruginosa* and *Staphylococcus aureus* 237 and 235 days, respectively, after injury. Those bacteria are associated with chronic complications (deep-wound infections and osteomyelitis), and it is not clear when they were introduced into the wounds. Limitations of the study include the small number of patients, the definitions available for defining extremity infections, and the fact that the JTTR has undergone changes in data collection methods that may have led to inconsistencies in the data.

Mody et al. (2009) assessed infections in 58 service members who had open or closed tibial or femoral fractures that culminated in intramedullary fixation and who were sent to WRAMC from October 2003 to June 2007. About 65% were IED-associated injuries. The authors reviewed inpatient and outpatient electronic health records and long-term followup (median, 447 days) was conducted with telephone interviews. Infectious complications occurred in 23 (40%) of the 58 patients. Osteomyelitits and hardware-associated infections were most common, occurring in 10 (43%) of 23 infected fractures (44%), or 17% of the total study populations. IED-associated injury was significantly more likely to be associated with infected fractures (21 of 23, 91%) than with noninfected fractures (17 of

35, 49%) (p = 0.005). Polymicrobial infections were common (occurring in 44% of infected fractures). Infecting bacteria were *Acinetobacter baumannii*, *Staphylococcus* species, MDR *Enterobacter cloacae*, and MDR *Klebsiella pneumoniae*.

Stevens et al. (1988) reported a case of a Vietnam veteran who sustained blast injuries from a land-mine explosion in 1967, developed gas gangrene that required amputation of his legs and several fingers, and then 17 years later had another episode of gas gangrene in a closed wound in his hand. *Clostridium perfringens* was cultured from the wound site. The patient was treated with penicillin, and no recurrence of infection was found at 6-month followup.

There is growing evidence that infections increase the risk of long-term cognitive decline. Shah et al. (2013) showed that there was a significant increase in the rates of cognitive impairment after pneumonia. That study of older Americans (mean age, 72.8 years) carefully controlled for patients' preinfection cognitive function and the trajectory of that function. The result reinforces similar findings that showed that severe sepsis was associated with an absolute increase of nearly 10 percentage points in the risk of moderate to severe cognitive impairment and a similarly dramatic increase in rates of disability (Iwashyna et al., 2010). Both those studies suggest that the cognitive declines were not limited to those who were most severely ill. The data are consistent with data from other studies that showed that modest levels of systemic inflammation—such as might occur with an infection treated in the outpatient setting—are associated with more rapid decline in patients with Alzheimer disease (Holmes et al., 2009). The possibility that blast-associated infections lead to such enduring cognitive declines has not been adequately studied. All the above studies included older patients, so the generalizability of their results to the younger military population is unknown.

## Conclusion

Various bacterial and fungal infections can occur after injury from exposure to blast, and multiple infections can occur in a single person. The infections can persist for days to months. Chronic infection also can lead to a state of sustained systemic inflammation with adverse long-term consequences for many organ systems. On the basis of the committee's expert clinical knowledge, it is plausible that infections related to blast injury can have long-term outcomes, including osteomyelitis, deep-wound infection, amputation, and delayed union.

**The committee concludes, on the basis of its evaluation, that there is inadequate/insufficient evidence of an association between exposure to blast and long-term effects of infections.**

## BURNS

Although burns are frequent after exposure to blast, few studies have assessed their outcomes, particularly long-term outcomes. The outcomes most often reported are length of hospital stay, gross functional outcomes, and mortality.

Four studies reported burn-patient outcomes at the US Army Institute of Surgical Research (USAISR) in San Antonio, Texas, which is the only US military burn center. Civilians from southern Texas can be treated there as well. From March 2003 to May 2005, Kauvar et al. (2006a) tracked 171 combat casualties of the Iraq and Afghanistan wars, of whom 119 (69.6%) were burned by IEDs and another 26.7% by conventional munitions. The combat casualties were compared with 102 patients (also military personnel) who received their burns from noncombat incidents involving, for example, burning of waste, ammunition and gunpowder mishaps, and misuse of gasoline. Most patients burned in explosions had burns to the hands and face. No difference was found between combat and noncombat patients in the length of stay at the burn center. However, combat patients generally spent more days in the intensive care unit (p = 0.08) and spent significantly more days using mechanical ventilation (p = 0.05). The overall mortality rate in both groups was low, but the mortality rate was higher in the combat patients than the noncombat patients, although there were too few patients to determine statistical significance. The vast majority of both groups (90.6% of combat and 98% of noncombat patients) were discharged to their own care. Sixty-seven percent of combat patients and 55.6% of noncombat patients returned to military duty, although many of them had medical limitations that prevented them from performing certain military tasks.

Kauvar et al. (2006b) identified 274 patients admitted to USAISR from April 5, 2003, to April 23, 2005, through medical records. All patients were military personnel in the Iraq and Afghanistan wars. Of the 274 patients, 142 were exposed to blast when they were injured as a result of detonation of an explosive device. The hands and head were the most frequently burned parts of the body in these patients. The authors reported outcomes in 125 of the 142 patients (they excluded 17 of the patients from the further analysis because they were still hospitalized). Five of the 125 patients died. The length of stay of the surviving 120 patients at the burn center ranged from 2 to 154 days (median, 14 days). Nearly all (91%) of the surviving patients were discharged to their own or their families' care. Four patients needed inpatient care after discharge from USAISR. Nearly half the patients were able to return to duty, although 10% had some duty limitations as a result of their injuries. Some 21% of the patients were released from military service, and 28% had pending decisions about their ability to return to service. With respect to functional recovery, 109 patients (91%) were discharged at their previous level of global functioning, 8 had moderate disability but were able to care for themselves, and 3 were severely disabled and unable to care for themselves.

Wolf et al. (2006) compared records of military personnel of the Iraq and Afghanistan wars who had burn injuries with records of civilians who had burn injuries treated at the same facility. Data were collected from April 2003 to May 2005, and a total of 751 patients were included. Of the 751, 273 patients were injured during military operations; the number injured specifically by blast was not stated. When age-adjusted, the mortality was similar in the military and civilian groups. The military patients had longer stays in the hospital but no difference in length of stay between the ICU and time spent on a ventilator. Gross functional outcomes were good (that is, previous level of function in activities of daily living) in 94% of the civilian and 92% of the military patients, moderate (can care for oneself with occasional assistance) in 5% of the civilian and 6% of the military patients, and severe (needs assistance for daily living) in 1% of the civilian and 2% of the military patients.

Return to duty status was measured in 61 military personnel who were treated at USAISR for hand burns from March 2003 through June 2005 (Chapman et al., 2008). Almost all the patients (60) had thermal burns, and one had an electric burn. Impairment and disability were measured on discharge from inpatient care and during a followup outpatient visit less than 4 months later. Some 67% (41) of the patients were able to return to duty. The remaining patients were discharged from military service for medical reasons. Patients who were not able to return to duty had greater total body-surface-area burns ($p < 0.001$) and greater full-thickness total body-surface-area burns ($p = 0.002$) than the ones who could return to duty.

A fifth study assessed clinical records of patients who were admitted to 10 hospitals during 1997–2003 in Israel (Peleg et al., 2008): 219 patients who had burn injuries related to terrorist attacks, 6,546 patients who had burn injuries not related to terrorist attacks, and 2,228 patients who experienced a terrorist attack but were not burned. The patients who had burn injuries related to terrorist attacks had longer hospital stays (mean, 18.5 days) than the patients who had burn injuries only (11.1 days) and the patients who were not burned (9.5 days). ISSs showed that injuries sustained in terrorist attacks that also involved burns were more severe than injuries sustained in terrorist attacks that did not result in burns or burn injuries not related to terrorist attacks. In-hospital mortality in patients whose burn injuries were related to terrorist attacks and patients who experienced a terrorist attack but were not burned were similar (6.4% vs 6.6%, respectively). However, patients who had burn injuries not related to terrorist attacks had lower mortality (3.4%). The difference in mortality could be due to the presence of multidimensional injuries associated with terrorist attacks.

Clinically, burns are known to lead to long-term complications. On the basis of its expert clinical knowledge, the committee does not have a reason to believe that burns from exposure to blast are different from burns from non-blast sources except that blast-related burns may have debris embedded in exposed skin. A number of long-term complications have been reported in non-blast burned patients and include scarring (Lawrence et al., 2012; Zanni, 2012), contracture (Schneider and Qu, 2011; Zanni, 2012), heterotopic ossification (Nelson et al., 2012a; Potter et al., 2007), abdominal complications (Markell et al., 2009), thromboembolic complications (Harrington et al., 2001), pruritus (Zachariah et al., 2012), loss of vision (Wisse et al., 2010), neurologic effects (Schneider and Qu, 2011), and psychologic effects (McKibben et al., 2009; Wiechman, 2011).

**The committee concludes, on the basis of its evaluation, that there is limited/suggestive evidence of an association between exposure to blast and long-term complications from burns.**

## BLAST PROTECTION

Protective equipment has been developed to protect military personnel from injuries caused by exposure to blast and gun shots: body armor (or vests, which can have add-on equipment, such as groin and deltoid protectors and neck collars), helmets, eye protection (spectacles and goggles), and ear protection (earplugs and earmuffs). Blast-resistant vehicles are another form of protective equipment. The committee was asked to consider whether improvements in collective and personal blast protection are associated with diminished blast injuries.

Two types of body armor are in use by the US military: soft and hard (NRC, 2012). Soft body armor is made of several compositions of aramid fibers, known as Kevlar and Twaron fibers. Vests made of aramid fibers are designed to protect against low-velocity, low-energy bullets (for example, 9-mm or .38 caliber bullets) and against shrapnel resulting from explosions. Hard body armor contains high-performance polyethylene fibers, known as Spectra or Dyneema fibers, or a ceramic composite material. It is designed to protect against high-velocity threats, such as .30 caliber and .50 caliber rifle bullets. All helmet types used by the US military are made of Kevlar. Two of the helmets, the Personnel Armored System for Ground Troops helmet and the Modular Integrated Communications helmet, are not sufficient to protect against TBI to an acceptable extent (McEntire and Whitely, 2005). The Advanced Combat Helmet met both the mean and peak standards for all impact experiments at an impact speed of 10 ft/s.

Greater detail about the composition of body armor and helmets is beyond the scope of this report, but further information can be found in Chapter 2 of the National Research Council's (NRC's) report *Testing of Body Armor Materials: Phase III* (2012).

In the past, the use of protective equipment has meant an overwhelming weight burden and the loss of dexterity and hand–eye coordination to the detriment of the render-safe mission (Bass et al., 2005). Even today, military personnel often opt not to wear protective equipment, because it can be uncomfortable and heavy, increase thermal burden, impede their ability to maneuver, and reduce situational awareness (Barwood et al., 2009; Breeze et al., 2012; Caldwell et al., 2011; Killion et al., 2011; Larsen et al., 2011; US Army, 2010). Protective equipment also may contribute to chronic health conditions, such as low-back pain (Burton et al., 1996; Konitzer et al., 2008). Indeed, the hard type of body armor can add a substantial burden of weight on military personnel. For example, the Improved Outer Tactical Vest Generation II body armor system can weigh 27.06–42.50 lb, depending on size (US Army, 2010). Given the main purpose of the body armor—to provide protection but still allow military personnel adequate mobility and flexibility—newer materials that have greater protective capabilities and are lighter are being continuously tested to improve protection.

Before being introduced in the field, protective equipment is tested to ensure that it meets military and law-enforcement standards. For gunshot and projectile injuries, the assessment methods include animal tests and "the correlation of animal chest deformation response with the response of simulant materials at velocities that are typical of rounds used to test soft body armors" (NRC, 2012, p. 34). For that type of assessment, gelatin is typically used as a tissue simulant; clay also can be used. Additional information about body armor standards and testing for gunshot and projectile injuries can be found in Chapter 3 of the NRC report mentioned above. Such a comprehensive set of guidelines does not exist for blast injuries. Nevertheless, in 2001, the North Atlantic Treaty Organization Research Technology Organization established a new task force, HFM-089/TG-024, to review how various countries test protective equipment against antipersonnel mines and their two main effects: fragmentation and blast (NATO, 2004). Among the recommendations of the task force were to use anthropomorphic mannequins to obtain good fit of protective equipment and Hybrid III anthropomorphic mannequins to perform blast tests against the upper body, including the head. The recommendations also emphasized the need for suitable instrumentation for the head, neck, and chest at a minimum and for reproducing militarily relevant conditions (using explosive charges and positioning the mannequins to mimic in-theater scenarios). Taking those recommendations into account, Bass et al. (2005) performed experiments on the effectiveness of body armor and helmets by using a 50th-percentile male Hybrid III anthropomorphic (automobile crash-test) dummy (First Technology Safety Systems, Inc., USA) exposed to a blast generated by detonating C4 charges of differing weights. The results showed the importance of acceleration and deceleration in neck and head injury although the study was limited by the type of instrumentation, which could measure only acceleration, not pressure. The authors concluded that the larger helmet and visor frontal surface areas tend to increase the risk of head injury from IED blasts owing to increased acceleration from increased exposure to the blast flow. However, the authors also concluded that the greater helmet mass tended to *decrease* the risk of head injury by decreasing the acceleration of the head, helmet, and visor system. The authors discussed the implications of their findings—either decreasing the visor area or increasing the mass of the helmet visor system or some combination of both increases should be implemented to achieve better protection from blunt trauma to the head. Nevertheless, careful consideration should be given to the facts that increasing the helmet mass without regard for ergonomic factors of wearability and comfort may decrease use of the head protection and lead to chronic neck microinjuries and that decreasing the visor and helmet size may make wearers more vulnerable to penetrating fragments (Bass et al., 2005). Despite the usefulness of those findings, the data are limited to protection from secondary and tertiary blast effects, not primary blasts.

The committee identified few studies of the effectiveness of protective equipment after introduction into the field. Belmont et al. (2010) reported that the percentage of military personnel killed in action in the Iraq and Afghanistan wars is similar to percentages in previous conflicts despite improvements in personal protective equipment and blast-resistant vehicles. The widespread use of explosive weaponry, including IEDs, in Iraq and Afghanistan shifted the etiology of military injuries from gunshot-induced to blast-induced, in contrast with previous wars. Thus, although the current body armor showed great success in reducing blunt and penetrating types of injuries because of its interceptive properties, it does not protect from or substantially reduce the damaging effects of primary blasts.

Breeze et al. (2011) conducted a systematic analysis of studies to assess whether face, neck, and eye protection affects the incidence of injuries in military personnel in the 21st century. In the identified studies, facial wounds had an incidence of 8–20%, neck wounds 2–11%, and eye wounds less than 1% to 6%. Use of eye protection was associated with a reduction by one-third in the rate of eye injuries in military personnel serving in Iraq and Afghanistan. When military personnel were in 100% compliance with the use of eye protection in Iraq, the incidence of eye injuries dropped from 6% to 0.5%. Breeze et al. (2012) assessed the effectiveness of neck protection (nape protectors and neck collars) in reducing the incidence of neck injuries. They identified, from the UK JTTR, neck wounds sustained by UK military personnel from January 1, 2006, to December 31, 2010. The incidence of neck wounds was 10% (152 of 1,528 injuries), and these wounds were more often caused by explosive events (79%) than by gun shots (21%). The records of 58% of those wounded stated whether they wore neck protection at the time of injury; all of those records indicated that they were not wearing neck protection. Of the 152 military personnel who had neck wounds, 111 (73%) died from the wounds. On the basis of the underlying pathology of the injuries and mapping the surface location of the neck injuries, the authors concluded that 16 of those deaths could have been prevented if neck collars had been worn. Eye protection was assessed in an additional study, although it is not specific for protection from exposure to blast. Thomas et al. (2009) assessed the effectiveness of combat eye protection in US service members deployed to the Iraq and Afghanistan wars. Using JTTR data on service members who entered level III hospital facilities from March 2003 to September 2006, the authors determined that eye injuries were significantly more frequent when person- nel did not wear eye protection ($p < 0.01$).

Several studies have evaluated the effectiveness of hearing protection in military personnel, although the studies focus on noise in general and not specifically on blast. A study of 449 cases of acute acoustic trauma in a military hospital in Helsinki, Finland, from 1989 to 1993 found that 14% of the cases had been using ear protection but one-third of them had poorly fitting protectors or insufficient protection (Savolainen and Lehtomaki, 1997). The IOM evaluated hearing-conservation programs in the military and reported that there was "limited or suggestive evidence to conclude that use of hearing protection devices and the level of real-world hearing protection these devices provide have been and remain not adequate in military hearing conservation programs" (IOM, 2006, p. 12). Casali et al. (2009) field-tested three hearing-enhancement protection systems (the Combat Arms Earplug, the Communication and Enhancement Protection System, and the Peltor Comtac II headset) in cadet soldier trainees in training exercises and found that improved hearing protection would be needed to obtain adequate levels of hearing performance for user compli- ance in the combat environment. Another study of hearing performance in people wearing hearing protection (the Combat Arms Earplug and the Sonic II Ear valves) reported that service members subject to high-level impulse noise would not experience compromised speech understanding when using level-dependent earplugs in low-level continuous noise (Norin et al., 2011). Finally, in a controlled field experiment that compared four hearing-protection enhancement devices (Peltor Com-Trac II, Etymotic EB1 and EB15 High-Fidelity Electronic BlastPLG electronic earplugs, and the 3M Single-Ended Combat Arms passive earplug) with the unprotected ear with ambient outdoor noise and in 82 dBA military diesel heavy-truck noise, none of the tested devices allowed normal localization performance.

Several studies have commented on whether the use of Kevlar body armor reduces the incidence of GU injury in battlefield combatants. A review of the changing patterns of wartime GU injuries in the preceding 100 years found a lower percentage of GU injuries that were abdominal in service members who wore body armor than in those service members who did not wear body armor (Hudak et al., 2005). The finding came primarily from a comparison of GU injuries in the 1991 Gulf War with those in the conflicts in Bosnia-Herzegovina. A review of 30 GU injuries in the 1991 Gulf War (body armor was worn) found that only 17% of the patients had abdominal GU injuries (Thompson et al., 1998), whereas in the Bosnian conflict (body armor was not worn) 45–53% of patients who had GU injuries had abdominal GU injuries (Hudolin and Hudolin, 2003). However, a more compressive evaluation of GU trauma of US service members who wore body armor (Serkin et al., 2010) showed that the percentage of abdominal GU trauma (kidney, ureter, and bladder) was 46.9%, which is quite similar to the percentage of abdominal GU trauma in the conflicts of Bosnia-Herzegovina. The percentage of these GU injuries in the conflicts of Bosnia-Herzegovina caused by blast (mostly from land mines and mortar and shell rounds) ranged from 52% to 70% (Vuckovic et al., 1995) and was similar to the percentage of GU injuries caused by blasts in Iraq and Afghanistan (50–63%) (Paquette, 2007; Serkin et al., 2010). However, the pattern of blast injuries in Iraq and Afghanistan caused by IEDs may be quite different from the pattern of blast injuries in Bosnia-Herzegovina caused by land mines and mortar shells, so comparing the protective effects of body armor related to GU trauma in different conflicts may have too many confounding factors. A retrospective review of GU trauma in the Iraq war found that US casualties who wore body armor had a significantly lower rate of GU injury than casualties who did not wear body armor (primarily Iraqi service members or civilians). Casualties who wore body armor had a 2.1% rate (25 of 1,216) of GU injury (upper and lower GU tract combined) versus 3.4% (51 of 1,496) in those who did not wear body armor (p = 0.037). Casualties who wore body armor had a 0.6% rate (7 of 1,216) rate of kidney injury versus 1.5% (22 of 1,496) in those who did not wear body armor (p = 0.017) (Paquette, 2007). The report seems to suggest that wearing protective body armor decreases the incidence of overall GU trauma and more specifically kidney injury. In light of the fact that most of the blast-induced GU injuries were caused by secondary blast effects (that is, shrapnel and particles of the environment generated during the explosion), the protective effects of the body armor are most probably due to its interceptive properties.

Laboratory testing can provide helpful information about the protective effects of body armor, although the current literature contains much controversial information. Although a study comparing the protective effects of two types of vests—one a soft protective vest and the other a hard protective vest—found that the vests significantly decreased pulmonary-injury risk after blast delivered via a shock tube (Wood et al., 2012), another study had opposite findings (Phillips et al., 1988). The latter study used sheep fitted with cloth ballistic vests and exposed to blasts with peak pressures of 115, 230, 295, and 420 kPa. It showed a significantly higher lung–body weight index (p < 0.05) than in sheep without vests; this suggested substantial lung edema (Phillips et al., 1988). At the highest exposure level (420 kPa), two of the six sheep without vests died and five of the six sheep with vests died. The authors concluded that the vests increased the target surface area and thus diminished the effective loading function on the thorax. It has been suggested that even minor displacements of the body wall may produce serious injury if the body wall velocity is high (Cooper and Taylor, 1989). Cooper et al. (1991) hypothesized that the motion of the body wall generates waves that propagate within the body and transfer energy to internal sites. Wave propagation has been identified as one of the essential mechanisms in the production of injuries resulting from blast impact to the torso, and mechanistic implications for effective personal protection from the primary effects of blast overpressure have been stressed (Cooper et al., 1991). Accordingly, it has been suggested that using a body armor developed on the basis of acoustic decoupling principles might reduce the direct stress coupled into the body and thus lessen the severity of lung injury. Li et al. (2006) reported that the ear barrel and ear plug showed protective effects against blast-induced trauma in the auditory organs of guinea pigs. Sheep and pigs placed in light-armor vehicles and exposed to blast showed more middle ear damage compared to control animals; no differences were found in the respiratory or gastrointestinal tracts (Phillips et al., 1989).

Ramasamy et al. (2011) assessed the effects of modifications of armored vehicles (V-shaped hull, increased ground clearance, widened axles, heavy vehicles, and blast deflectors) used during the Rhodesian War (1972–1980) on rates of injury. Data were available on 2,212 vehicle–mine incidents involving 16,456 people. All the vehicle modifications statistically significantly reduced fatality rates and they had a cumulative effect. Except for blast deflectors, they also reduced injury rates. As in personal protective equipment, the modifications of the vehicles probably reduced the amount of energy transferred to and interacting directly with the service members' bodies.

The importance of correctly fitting personal protective equipment cannot be overestimated. Anecdotal data indicate that body armor that is too small or too large might increase the injurious effects of a blast via enhancement of the impact-related parenchymal organ damage or via reflection of refraction waves from the body wall and inside body armor that amplify the shock wave coupling with the body. Nevertheless, further well-designed studies that use standardized and militarily relevant models are needed to clarify the mechanisms underlying the negative side effects caused by the ill fit of personal protective equipment.

The committee concludes, on the basis of its evaluation, that there is sufficient evidence of an association between the use of personal protective equipment, including interceptive body armor and eye protection, and prevention of blunt and penetrating injuries caused by exposure to blast.

The committee concludes, on the basis of its evaluation, that there is inadequate/insufficient evidence to determine whether an association exists between the use of current personal protective equipment and prevention of primary blast-induced (non-impact-induced) injuries.

## REFERENCES

ACRM (American Congress of Rehabilitation Medicine). 1993. Definition of mild traumatic brain injury. *Journal of Head Trauma Rehabilitation* 8(3):86-87.

Alam, M., M. Iqbal, A. Khan, and S. A. Khan. 2012. Ocular injuries in blast victims. *Journal of the Pakistan Medical Association* 62(2):138-142.

Albrecht, M. C., M. E. Griffith, C. K. Murray, K. K. Chung, E. E. Horvath, J. A. Ward, D. R. Hospenthal, J. B. Holcomb, and S. E. Wolf. 2006. Impact of acinetobacter infection on the mortality of burn patients. *Journal of the American College of Surgeons* 203(4):546-550.

Aldrich, T. K., J. Gustave, C. B. Hall, H. W. Cohen, M. P. Webber, R. Zeig-Owens, K. Cosenza, V. Christodoulou, L. Glass, F. Al-Othman, M. D. Weiden, K. J. Kelly, and D. J. Prezant. 2010. Lung function in rescue workers at the World Trade Center after 7 years. *New England Journal of Medicine* 362(14):1263-1272.

Alexander, M. P. 1995. Mild traumatic brain injury: Pathophysiology, natural-history, and clinical management. *Neurology* 45(7):1253-1260.

Alfieri, K. A., J. Forsberg, and B. K. Potter. 2012. Blast injuries and heterotopic ossification. *Bone and Joint Research* 1(8):192-197.

Andelic, N., N. Hammergren, E. Bautz-Holter, U. Sveen, C. Brunborg, and C. Roe. 2009. Functional outcome and health-related quality of life 10 years after moderate-to-severe traumatic brain injury. *Acta Neurologica Scandinavica* 120(1):16-23.

Andersen, R. C., M. Fleming, J. A. Forsberg, W. T. Gordon, G. P. Nanos, M. T. Charlton, and J. R. Ficke. 2012. Dismounted complex blast injury. *Journal of Surgical Orthopaedic Advances* 21(1):2-7.

APA (American Psychiatric Association). 2013. *Diagnostic and Statistical Manual for Mental Disorders.* 5th ed. Washington, DC: American Psychiatric Publishing.

Argyros, G. J. 1997. Management of primary blast injury. *Toxicology* 121(1):105-115

Armonda, R. A., R. S. Bell, A. H. Vo, G. Ling, T. J. DeGraba, B. Crandall, J. Ecklund, and W. W. Campbell. 2006. Wartime traumatic cerebral vasospasm: Recent review of combat casualties. *Neurosurgery* 59(6):1215-1225.

Avidan, V., M. Hersch, Y. Armon, R. Spira, D. Aharoni, P. Reissman, and W. P. Schecter. 2005. Blast lung injury: Clinical manifestations, treatment, and outcome. *American Journal of Surgery* 190(6):927-931.

Barros D'Sa, A. A. B., T. H. Hassard, R. H. Livingston, and J. W. S. Irwin. 1980. Missile-induced vascular trauma. *Injury* 12(1):13-30.

Barwood, M. J., P. S. Newton, and M. J. Tipton. 2009. Ventilated vest and tolerance for intermittent exercise in hot, dry conditions with military clothing. *Aviation Space & Environmental Medicine* 80(4):353-359.

Bass, C. R., M. Davis, K. Rafaels, M. S. Rountree, R. M. Harris, E. Sanderson, W. Andrefsky, G. DiMarco, and M. Zielinski. 2005. A methodology for assessing blast protection in explosive ordnance disposal bomb suits. *International Journal of Occupational Safety & Ergonomics* 11(4):347-361.

Baxter, D., D. J. Sharp, C. Feeney, D. Papadopoulou, T. E. Ham, S. Jilka, P. J. Hellyer, M. C. Patel, A. N. Bennett, A. Mistlin, E. McGilloway, M. Midwinter, and A. P. Goldstone. 2013. Pituitary dysfunction after blast traumatic brain injury: UK biosap study. *Annals of Neurology* 74(4):527-536.

Bazarian, J. J., K. Donnelly, D. R. Peterson, G. C. Warner, T. Zhu, and J. Zhong. 2013. The relation between posttraumatic stress disorder and mild traumatic brain injury acquired during Operations Enduring Freedom and Iraqi Freedom. *Journal of Head Trauma Rehabilitation* 28(1):1-12.

Bell, R. S., A. H. Vo, C. J. Neal, J. Tigno, R. Roberts, C. Mossop, J. R. Dunne, and R. A. Armonda. 2009. Military traumatic brain and spinal column injury: A 5-year study of the impact blast and other military grade weaponry on the central nervous system. *The Journal of Trauma* 66(4 Suppl):S104-S111.

Belmont, P. J., Jr., G. P. Goodman, M. Zacchilli, M. Posner, C. Evans, and B. D. Owens. 2010. Incidence and epidemiology of combat injuries sustained during "the Surge" portion of Operation Iraqi Freedom by a U.S. Army brigade combat team. *Journal of Trauma: Injury, Infection, & Critical Care* 68(1):204-210.

Bennett, J. W., J. L. Robertson, D. R. Hospenthal, S. E. Wolf, K. K. Chung, K. Mende, and C. K. Murray. 2010. Impact of extended spectrum beta-lactamase producing klebsiella pneumoniae infections in severely burned patients. *Journal of the American College of Surgeons* 211(3):391-399.

Blair, J. A., J. C. Patzkowski, A. J. Schoenfeld, J. D. Cross Rivera, E. S. Grenier, R. A. Lehman, Jr., and J. R. Hsu. 2012. Spinal column injuries among Americans in the global war on terrorism. *Journal of Bone and Joint Surgery—American Volume* 94(18):e135(131-139).

Blanch, R. J., M. S. Bindra, A. S. Jacks, and R. A. H. Scott. 2011. Ophthalmic injuries in British armed forces in Iraq and Afghanistan. *Eye* 25(2):218-223.

Brahm, K. D., H. M. Wilgenburg, J. Kirby, S. Ingalla, C.-Y. Chang, and G. L. Goodrich. 2009. Visual impairment and dysfunction in combat-injured service members with traumatic brain injury. *Optometry & Vision Science* 86(7):817-825.

Breeze, J., I. Horsfall, A. Hepper, and J. Clasper. 2011. Face, neck, and eye protection: Adapting body armour to counter the changing patterns of injuries on the battlefield. *British Journal of Oral and Maxillofacial Surgery* 49(8):602-606.

Breeze, J., L. S. Allanson-Bailey, N. C. Hunt, R. S. Delaney, A. E. Hepper, and J. Clasper. 2012. Mortality and morbidity from combat neck injury. *The Journal of Trauma and Acute Care Surgery* 72(4):969-974.

Brenner, L. A., N. Bahraini, and T. D. Hernandez. 2012. Perspectives on creating clinically relevant blast models for mild traumatic brain injury and post traumatic stress disorder symptoms. *Frontiers in Neurology [electronic resource]* 3:31.

Breyer, B., B. Cohen, D. Berterthal, R. Rosen, T. Neylan, and K. Seal. 2012. The association of posttraumatic stress disorder with lower urinary tract symptoms in male Iraq and Afghanistan veterans. *Journal of Urology* 187(4):e696.

Brown, K. V., C. K. Murray, and J. C. Clasper. 2010. Infectious complications of combat-related mangled extremity injuries in the British military. *Journal of Trauma: Injury, Infection, & Critical Care* 69(Suppl 1):S109-S115.

Bryant, R. A., M. Creamer, M. O'Donnell, D. Silove, C. R. Clark, and A. C. McFarlane. 2009. Post-traumatic amnesia and the nature of post-traumatic stress disorder after mild traumatic brain injury. *Journal of the International Neuropsychological Society* 15(6):862-867.

Burton, A. K., K. M. Tillotson, T. L. Symonds, C. Burke, and T. Mathewson. 1996. Occupational risk factors for the first-onset and subsequent course of low back trouble. A study of serving police officers. *Spine* 21(22):2612-2620.

Caldwell, J. N., L. Engelen, C. van der Henst, M. J. Patterson, and N. A. Taylor. 2011. The interaction of body armor, low-intensity exercise, and hot-humid conditions on physiological strain and cognitive function. *Military Medicine* 176(5):488-493.

Calvano, T. P., D. R. Hospenthal, E. M. Renz, S. E. Wolf, and C. K. Murray. 2010. Central nervous system infections in patients with severe burns. *Burns* 36(5):688-691.

Capo-Aponte, J. E., T. G. Urosevich, L. A. Temme, A. K. Tarbett, and N. K. Sanghera. 2012. Visual dysfunctions and symptoms during the subacute stage of blast-induced mild traumatic brain injury. *Military Medicine* 177(7):804-813.

Carpenter, R. J., J. D. Hartzell, J. A. Forsberg, B. S. Babel, and A. Ganesan. 2008. Pseudomonas putida war wound infection in a US marine: A case report and review of the literature. *Journal of Infection* 56(4):234-240.

Casali, J. G., W. A. Ahroon, and J. A. Lancaster. 2009. A field investigation of hearing protection and hearing enhancement in one device: For soldiers whose ears and lives depend upon it. *Noise Health* 11(42):69-90.

Caseby, N. G., and M. F. Porter. 1976. Blast injuries to the lungs: Clinical presentation, management and course. *Injury* 8(1):1-12.

CDC (Centers for Disease Control and Prevention). 2008a. *Blast Injuries: Abdominal Blast Injuries.* http://www.bt.cdc.gov/masscasualties/blastinjury-abdominal.asp (accessed March 1, 2013).

CDC. 2008b. *Blast Injuries: Blast Extremity Injuries.* http://www.bt.cdc.gov/masscasualties/blastinjury-extremity.asp (accessed March 1, 2013).

CDC. 2010. *Blast Injuries: Crush Injuries and Crush Syndrome.* http://www.bt.cdc.gov/masscasualties/blastinjury-crush.asp (accessed March 1, 2013).

CDC. 2012. *Blast Injuries: Blast Lung Injury.* http://www.bt.cdc.gov/masscasualties/blastlunginjury.asp (accessed March 1, 2013).

Champion, H. R., J. B. Holcomb, and L. A. Young. 2009. Injuries from explosions: Physics, biophysics, pathology, and required research focus. *Journal of Trauma: Injury, Infection, & Critical Care* 66(5):1468-1477; discussion 1477.

Chapman, T. T., R. L. Richard, T. L. Hedman, E. M. Renz, S. E. Wolf, and J. B. Holcomb. 2008. Combat casualty hand burns: Evaluating impairment and disability during recovery. *Journal of Hand Therapy* 21(2):150-158; quiz 159.

Cockerham, G. C., S. Lemke, C. Glynn-Milley, L. Zumhagen, and K. P. Cockerham. 2013. Visual performance and the ocular surface in traumatic brain injury. *The Ocular Surface* 11(1):25-34.

Coe, C. D., K. S. Bower, D. B. Brooks, R. D. Stutzman, and J. B. Hammer. 2010. Effect of blast trauma and corneal foreign bodies on visual performance. *Optometry & Vision Science* 87(8):604-611.

Cohen, J. T., G. Ziv, J. Bloom, D. Zikk, Y. Rapoport, and M. Z. Himmelfarb. 2002. Blast injury of the ear in a confined space explosion: Auditory and vestibular evaluation. *Israel Medical Association Journal* 4(7):559-562.

Coker, W. J., B. M. Bhatt, N. F. Blatchley, and J. T. Graham. 1999. Clinical findings for the first 1000 Gulf War veterans in the Ministry of Defence's medical assessment programme. *British Medical Journal* 318(7179):290-294.

Coldren, R. L., M. L. Russell, R. V. Parish, M. Dretsch, and M. P. Kelly. 2012. The ANAM lacks utility as a diagnostic or screening tool for concussion more than 10 days following injury. *Military Medicine* 177(2):179-183.

Comstock, S., D. Pannell, M. Talbot, L. Compton, N. Withers, and H. C. Tien. 2011. Spinal injuries after improvised explosive device incidents: Implications for tactical combat casualty care. *Journal of Trauma: Injury, Infection, & Critical Care* 71(5 Suppl 1):S413-S417.

Cooper, D. B., P. M. Chau, P. Armistead-Jehle, R. D. Vanderploeg, and A. O. Bowles. 2012. Relationship between mechanism of injury and neurocognitive functioning in OEF/OIF service members with mild traumatic brain injuries. *Military Medicine* 177(10):1157-1160.

Cooper, G. J., and D. E. Taylor. 1989. Biophysics of impact injury to the chest and abdomen. *Journal of the Royal Army Medical Corps* 135(2):58-67.

Cooper, G. J., R. L. Maynard, N. L. Cross, and J. F. Hill. 1983. Casualties from terrorist bombings. *Journal of Trauma: Injury, Infection, & Critical Care* 23(11):955-967.

Cooper, G. J., D. J. Townend, S. R. Cater, and B. P. Pearce. 1991. The role of stress waves in thoracic visceral injury from blast loading: Modification of stress transmission by foams and high-density materials. *Journal of Biomechanics* 24(5):273-285.

Couch, J. R., R. B. Lipton, W. F. Stewart, and A. I. Scher. 2007. Head or neck injury increases the risk of chronic daily headache: A population-based study. *Neurology* 69(11):1169-1177.

Covey, D. C. 2002. Blast and fragment injuries of the musculoskeletal system. *Journal of Bone & Joint Surgery—American Volume* 84(7):1221-1234.

Coy, J., and G. Chatfield. 1998. Bilateral total knee replacement for traumatic arthritis from blast injury in Vietnam. *Military Medicine* 163(9):651-652.

Cross, J. D., D. J. Stinner, T. C. Burns, J. C. Wenke, and J. R. Hsu. 2012. Return to duty after type III open tibia fracture. *Journal of Orthopaedic Trauma* 26(1):43-47.

Cuthbertson, B. H., S. Roughton, D. Jenkinson, G. Maclennan, and L. Vale. 2010. Quality of life in the five years after intensive care: A cohort study. *Critical Care (London, England)* 14(1):R6.

Dau, B., G. Oda, and M. Holodniy. 2009. Infectious complications in OIF/OEF veterans with traumatic brain injury. *Journal of Rehabilitation Research & Development* 46(6):673-684.

Davenport, N. D., K. O. Lim, M. T. Armstrong, and S. R. Sponheim. 2012. Diffuse and spatially variable white matter disruptions are associated with blast-related mild traumatic brain injury. *Neuroimage* 59(3):2017-2024.

D'Avignon, L. C., B. K. Hogan, C. K. Murray, F. L. Loo, D. R. Hospenthal, L. C. Cancio, S. H. Kim, E. M. Renz, D. Barillo, J. B. Holcomb, C. E. Wade, and S. E. Wolf. 2010. Contribution of bacterial and viral infections to attributable mortality in patients with severe burns: An autopsy series. *Burns* 36(6):773-779.

DePalma, R. G., D. G. Burris, H. R. Champion, and M. J. Hodgson. 2005. Blast injuries. *New England Journal of Medicine* 352(13):1335-1342.

Desai, S. V., T. J. Law, and D. M. Needham. 2011. Long-term complications of critical care. *Critical Care Medicine* 39(2):371-379.

DOD (Department of Defense). 2007. *Mental Health Encounters and Diagnoses Following Deployment to Iraq and/or Afghanistan, U.S. Armed forces, 2001-2006.* http://www.afhsc.mil/viewMSMR?file=2007/v14_n04.pdf (accessed July 14, 2013).

Dougherty, P. J. 1999. Long-term followup study of bilateral above-the-knee amputees from the Vietnam War. *Journal of Bone & Joint Surgery—American Volume* 81(10):1384-1390.

Eardley, W. G. P., T. J. Bonner, I. E. Gibb, and J. C. Clasper. 2012. Spinal fractures in current military deployments. *Journal of the Royal Army Medical Corps* 158(2):101-105.

Eastridge, B. J., R. L. Mabry, P. Seguin, J. Cantrell, T. Tops, P. Uribe, O. Mallett, T. Zubko, L. Oetjen-Gerdes, T. E. Rasmussen, F. K. Butler, R. S. Kotwal, J. B. Holcomb, C. Wade, H. Champion, M. Lawnick, L. Moores, and L. H. Blackbourne. 2012. Death on the battlefield (2001-2011): Implications for the future of combat casualty care. *Journal of Trauma and Acute Care Surgery* 73:S431-S437.

Eckert, M. J., C. Clagett, M. Martin, and K. Azarow. 2006. Bronchoscopy in the blast injury patient. *Archives of Surgery* 141(8):806-809; discussion 806-811.

Ersoz, M., K. Kaya, S. Akkus, and S. Ozel. 2011. Urodynamic findings in patients with traumatic brain injury. *Turkiye Fiziksel Tip ve Rehabilitasyon Dergisi* 57(2):80-84.

Fasol, R., S. Irvine, and P. Zilla. 1989. Vascular injuries caused by anti-personnel mines. *Journal of Cardiovascular Surgery (Torino)* 30(3):467-472.

Feldt, B. A., N. L. Salinas, T. E. Rasmussen, and J. Brennan. 2013. The joint facial and invasive neck trauma (J-FAINT) project, Iraq and Afghanistan 2003-2011. *Otolaryngology—Head & Neck Surgery* 148(3):403-408.

Finlay, S. E., M. Earby, D. J. Baker, and V. S. G. Murray. 2012. Explosions and human health: The long-term effects of blast injury. *Prehospital and Disaster Medicine* 27(4):385-391.

Fischer, H. 2013. U.S. Military Casualty Statistics: Operation New Dawn, Operation Iraqi Freedom, and Operation Enduring Freedom. RS22452 Congressional Research Service.

Fleming, M., S. Waterman, J. Dunne, J.-C. D'Alleyrand, and R. C. Andersen. 2012. Dismounted complex blast injuries: Patterns of injuries and resource utilization associated with the multiple extremity amputee. *Journal of Surgical Orthopaedic Advances* 21(1):32-37.

Forsberg, J. A., J. M. Pepek, S. Wagner, K. Wilson, J. Flint, R. C. Andersen, D. Tadaki, F. A. Gage, A. Stojadinovic, and E. A. Elster. 2009. Heterotopic ossification in high-energy wartime extremity injuries: Prevalence and risk factors. *Journal of Bone & Joint Surgery—American Volume* 91(5):1084-1091.

Gallun, F. J., A. C. Diedesch, L. R. Kubli, T. C. Walden, R. L. Folmer, M. S. Lewis, D. J. McDermott, S. A. Fausti, and M. R. Leek. 2012a. Performance on tests of central auditory processing by individuals exposed to high-intensity blasts. *Journal of Rehabilitation Research & Development* 49(7):1005-1025.

Gallun, F. J., M. S. Lewis, R. L. Folmer, A. C. Diedesch, L. R. Kubli, D. J. McDermott, T. C. Walden, S. A. Fausti, H. L. Lew, and M. R. Leek. 2012b. Implications of blast exposure for central auditory function: A review. *Journal of Rehabilitation Research & Development* 49(7):1059-1074.

Ghosh, S. K., D. Bandyopadhyay, A. Ghosh, S. Sarkar, and R. K. Mandal. 2009. Prurigo nodularis-like skin eruptions after bomb-blast injury. *Clinical and Experimental Dermatology* 34(7):e471-472.

Giannantoni, A., D. Silvestro, S. Siracusano, E. Azicnuda, M. D'Ippolito, J. Rigon, U. Sabatini, V. Bini, and R. Formisano. 2011. Urologic dysfunction and neurologic outcome in coma survivors after severe traumatic brain injury in the postacute and chronic phase. *Archives of Physical Medicine & Rehabilitation* 92(7):1134-1138.

Goldstein, L. E., A. M. Fisher, C. A. Tagge, X. L. Zhang, L. Velisek, J. A. Sullivan, C. Upreti, J. M. Kracht, M. Ericsson, M. W. Wojnarowicz, C. J. Goletiani, G. M. Maglakelidze, N. Casey, J. A. Moncaster, O. Minaeva, R. D. Moir, C. J. Nowinski, R. A. Stern, R. C. Cantu, J. Geiling, J. K. Blusztajn, B. L. Wolozin, T. Ikezu, T. D. Stein, A. E. Budson, N. W. Kowall, D. Chargin, A. Sharon, S. Saman, G. F. Hall, W. C. Moss, R. O. Cleveland, R. E. Tanzi, P. K. Stanton, and A. C. McKee. 2012. Chronic traumatic encephalopathy in blast-exposed military veterans and a blast neurotrauma mouse model. *Science Translational Medicine* 4(134):1-16.

Goodrich, G. L., J. Kirby, G. Cockerham, S. P. Ingalla, and H. L. Lew. 2007. Visual function in patients of a polytrauma rehabilitation center: A descriptive study. *Journal of Rehabilitation Research & Development* 44(7):929-936.

Goodrich, G. L., H. M. Flyg, J. E. Kirby, C. Y. Chang, and G. L. Martinsen. 2013. Mechanisms of TBI and visual consequences in military and veteran populations. *Optometry and Vision Science* 90(2):105-112.

Harrington, D. T., D. W. Mozingo, L. Cancio, P. Bird, B. Jordan, and C. W. Goodwin. 2001. Thermally injured patients are at significant risk for thromboembolic complications. *Journal of Trauma: Injury, Infection, & Critical Care* 50(3):495-499.

Heltemes, K. J., T. L. Holbrook, A. J. Macgregor, and M. R. Galarneau. 2012. Blast-related mild traumatic brain injury is associated with a decline in self-rated health amongst US military personnel. *Injury* 43(12):1990-1995.

Heltemes, K. J., M. C. Clouser, A. J. Macgregor, S. B. Norman, and M. R. Galarneau. 2013. Co-occurring mental health and alcohol misuse: Dual disorder symptoms in combat injured veterans. *Addictive Behaviors* 39(2):392-398.

Herridge, M. S., C. M. Tansey, A. Matte, G. Tomlinson, N. Diaz-Granados, A. Cooper, C. B. Guest, C. D. Mazer, S. Mehta, T. E. Stewart, P. Kudlow, D. Cook, A. S. Slutsky, and A. M. Cheung. 2011. Functional disability 5 years after acute respiratory distress syndrome. *New England Journal of Medicine* 364(14):1293-1304.

Hicks, R. R., S. J. Fertig, R. E. Desrocher, W. J. Koroshetz, and J. J. Pancrazio. 2010. Neurological effects of blast injury. *Journal of Trauma: Injury, Infection, & Critical Care* 68(5):1257-1263.

Hilz, M. J., P. A. DeFina, S. Anders, J. Koehn, C. J. Lang, E. Pauli, S. R. Flanagan, S. Schwab, and H. Marthol. 2011. Frequency analysis unveils cardiac autonomic dysfunction after mild traumatic brain injury. *Journal of Neurotrauma* 28(9):1727-1738.

Hirshberg, B., A. Oppenheim-Eden, R. Pizov, M. Sklair-Levi, A. Rivkin, E. Bardach, M. Bublil, C. Sprung, and M. R. Kramer. 1999. Recovery from blast lung injury: One-year followup. *Chest* 116(6):1683-1688.

Hoge, C. W., J. C. Clark, and C. A. Castro. 2007. Commentary: Women in combat and the risk of post-traumatic stress disorder and depression. *International Journal of Epidemiology* 36(2):327-329.

Hoge, C. W., D. McGurk, J. L. Thomas, A. L. Cox, C. C. Engel, and C. A. Castro. 2008. Mild traumatic brain injury in U.S. soldiers returning from Iraq. *New England Journal of Medicine* 358(5):453-463.

Holmes, C., C. Cunningham, E. Zotova, J. Woolford, C. Dean, S. Kerr, D. Culliford, and V. H. Perry. 2009. Systemic inflammation and disease progression in Alzheimer disease. *Neurology* 73(10):768-774.

Horvath, E. E., C. K. Murray, G. M. Vaughan, K. K. Chung, D. R. Hospenthal, C. E. Wade, J. B. Holcomb, S. E. Wolf, A. D. Mason, Jr., and L. C. Cancio. 2007. Fungal wound infection (not colonization) is independently associated with mortality in burn patients. *Annals of Surgery* 245(6):978-985.

Hrubec, Z., and R. A. Ryder. 1980. Traumatic limb amputations and subsequent mortality from cardiovascular disease and other causes. *Journal of Chronic Diseases* 33(4):239-250.

Huang, M. X., S. Nichols, A. Robb, A. Angeles, A. Drake, M. Holland, S. Asmussen, J. D'Andrea, W. Chun, M. Levy, L. Cui, T. Song, D. G. Baker, P. Hammer, R. McLay, R. J. Theilmann, R. Coimbra, M. Diwakar, C. Boyd, J. Neff, T. T. Liu, J. Webb-Murphy, R. Farinpour, C. Cheung, D. L. Harrington, D. Heister, and R. R. Lee. 2012. An automatic MEG low-frequency source imaging approach for detecting injuries in mild and moderate TBI patients with blast and non-blast causes. *Neuroimage* 61(4):1067-1082.

Hudak, S. J., A. F. Morey, T. A. Rozanski, and C. W. Fox, Jr. 2005. Battlefield urogenital injuries: Changing patterns during the past century. *Urology* 65(6):1041-1046.

Hudolin, T., and I. Hudolin. 2003. Surgical management of urogenital injuries at a war hospital in Bosnia-Hrzegovina, 1992 to 1995. *Journal of Urology* 169(4):1357-1359.

Huller, T., and Y. Bazini. 1970. Blast injuries of the chest and abdomen. *Archives of Surgery* 100(1):24-30.

IOM (Institute of Medicine). 2006. *Noise and Military Service: Implications for Hearing Loss and Tinnitus.* Washington, DC: The National Academies Press.

IOM. 2009. *Gulf War and Health, Volume 7: Long-Term Consequences of Traumatic Brain Injury.* Washington, DC: The National Academies Press.

Iwashyna, T. J., E. W. Ely, D. M. Smith, and K. M. Langa. 2010. Long-term cognitive impairment and functional disability among survivors of severe sepsis. *Journal of the American Medical Association* 304(16):1787-1794.

Jagade, M. V., R. A. Patil, I. S. Suhail, P. Kelkar, S. Nemane, J. Mahendru, V. Kalbande, and P. Kewle. 2008. Bomb blast injury: Effect on middle and inner ear. *Indian Journal of Otolaryngology and Head and Neck Surgery* 60(4):324-330.

Johnson, E. N., T. C. Burns, R. A. Hayda, D. R. Hospenthal, and C. K. Murray. 2007a. Infectious complications of open type III tibial fractures among combat casualties. *Clinical Infectious Diseases* 45(4):409-415.

Johnson, I. O. N., C. J. Fox, P. White, E. Adams, M. Cox, N. Rich, and D. L. Gillespie. 2007b. Physical exam and occult post-traumatic vascular lesions: Implications for the evaluation and management of arterial injuries in modern warfare in the endovascular era. *Journal of Cardiovascular Surgery* 48(5):581-586.

Jorge, R. E., L. Acion, T. White, D. Tordesillas-Gutierrez, R. Pierson, B. Crespo-Facorro, and V. A. Magnotta. 2012. White matter abnormalities in veterans with mild traumatic brain injury. *American Journal of Psychiatry* 169(12):1284-1291.

Kauvar, D. S., L. C. Cancio, S. E. Wolf, C. E. Wade, and J. B. Holcomb. 2006a. Comparison of combat and non-combat burns from ongoing U.S. military operations. *Journal of Surgical Research* 132(2):195-200.

Kauvar, D. S., S. E. Wolf, C. E. Wade, L. C. Cancio, E. M. Renz, and J. B. Holcomb. 2006b. Burns sustained in combat explosions in Operations Iraqi and Enduring Freedom (OIF/OEF explosion burns). *Burns* 32(7):853-857.

Keen, E. F., 3rd, C. K. Murray, B. J. Robinson, D. R. Hospenthal, E. M. Co, and W. K. Aldous. 2010. Changes in the incidences of multidrug-resistant and extensively drug-resistant organisms isolated in a military medical center. *Infection Control and Hospital Epidemiology* 31(7):728-732.

Kelly, J. F., A. E. Ritenour, D. F. McLaughlin, K. A. Bagg, A. N. Apodaca, C. T. Mallak, L. Pearse, M. M. Lawnick, H. R. Champion, C. E. Wade, and J. B. Holcomb. 2008. Injury severity and causes of death from Operation Iraqi Freedom and Operation Enduring Freedom: 2003-2004 versus 2006. *Journal of Trauma: Injury, Infection, & Critical Care* 64(2 Suppl):S21-S26; discussion S26-S27.

Kennedy, J. E., M. A. Cullen, R. R. Amador, J. C. Huey, and F. O. Leal. 2010. Symptoms in military service members after blast mTBI with and without associated injuries. *Neurorehabilitation* 26(3):191-197.

Kessler, R. C., A. Sonnega, E. Bromet, M. Hughes, and C. B. Nelson. 1995. Posttraumatic-stress-disorder in the National Comorbidity Survey. *Archives of General Psychiatry* 52(12):1048-1060.

Kessler, R. C., P. Berglund, O. Demler, R. Jin, and E. E. Walters. 2005. Lifetime prevalence and age-of-onset distributions of DSM-IV disorders in the National Comorbidity Survey Replication. *Archives of General Psychiatry* 62(6):593-602.

Kessler, R. C., M. Petukhova, N. A. Sampson, A. M. Zaslavsky, and H.-U. Wittchen. 2012. Twelve-month and lifetime prevalence and lifetime morbid risk of anxiety and mood disorders in the United States. *International Journal of Methods in Psychiatric Research* 21(3):169-184.

Killion, M. C., T. Monroe, and V. Drambarean. 2011. Better protection from blasts without sacrificing situational awareness. *International Journal of Audiology* 50(Suppl 1): S38-S45.

King, M. S., J. E. Johnson, R. F. Miller, R. Eisenberg, J. H. Newman, J. J. Tolle, J. F. E. Harrell, H. Nian, M. Ninan, E. S. Lambright, and J. R. Sheller. 2011. Constrictive bronchiolitis in soldiers returning from Iraq and Afghanistan. *New England Journal of Medicine* 365(3):222-230.

Kishikawa, M., T. Yoshioka, T. Shimazu, H. Sugimoto, T. Yoshioka, and T. Sugimoto. 1991. Pulmonary contusion causes long-term respiratory dysfunction with decreased functional residual capacity. *Journal of Trauma* 31(9):1203-1210.

Koc, E., M. Tunca, A. Akar, A. H. Erbil, B. Demiralp, and E. Arca. 2008. Skin problems in amputees: A descriptive study. *International Journal of Dermatology* 47(5):463-466.

Konitzer, L. N., M. V. Fargo, T. L. Brininger, and M. Lim Reed. 2008. Association between back, neck, and upper extremity musculoskeletal pain and the individual body armor. *Journal of Hand Therapy* 21(2):143-148; quiz 149.

Krzywiecki, A., D. Ziora, G. Niepsuj, D. Jastrzebski, S. Dworniczak, and J. Kozielski. 2007. Late consequences of respiratory system burns. *Journal of Physiology & Pharmacology* 58(Suppl 5)(Pt 1):319-325.

Kushelevsky, B. P. 1949. Pulmonary emphysema combined with bronchial asthma following injury. *Klinicheskaia Meditsina* 27(3):3-10.

Larsen, B., K. Netto, and B. Aisbett. 2011. The effect of body armor on performance, thermal stress, and exertion: A critical review. *Military Medicine* 176(11):1265-1273.

Lawrence, J. W., S. T. Mason, K. Schomer, and M. B. Klein. 2012. Epidemiology and impact of scarring after burn injury: A systematic review of the literature. *Journal of Burn Care & Research* 33(1):136-146.

Leibovici, D., O. N. Gofrit, M. Stein, S. C. Shapira, Y. Noga, R. J. Heruti, and J. Shemer. 1996. Blast injuries: Bus versus open-air bombings: A comparative study of injuries in survivors of open-air versus confined-space explosions. *Journal of Trauma: Injury, Infection, & Critical Care* 41(6):1030-1035.

Leone, M., F. Brégeon, F. Antonini, K. Chaumoître, A. Charvet, L. H. Ban, Y. Jammes, J. Albanèse, and C. Martin. 2008. Long-term outcome in chest trauma. *Anesthesiology* 109(5):864-871.

Levin, H. S., E. Wilde, M. Troyanskaya, N. J. Petersen, R. Scheibel, M. Newsome, M. Radaideh, T. Wu, R. Yallampalli, Z. Chu, and X. Li. 2010. Diffusion tensor imaging of mild to moderate blast-related traumatic brain injury and its sequelae. *Journal of Neurotrauma* 27(4):683-694.

Lew, H. L., T. K. Pogoda, E. Baker, K. L. Stolzmann, M. Meterko, D. X. Cifu, J. Amara, and A. M. Hendricks. 2011. Prevalence of dual sensory impairment and its association with traumatic brain injury and blast exposure in OEF/OIF veterans. *Journal of Head Trauma Rehabilitation* 26(6):489-496.

Li, C.J., P.F. Zhu, Z.H. Liu, Z.G. Wang, C. Yang, H.B. Chen, X. Ning, J.H. Zhou, and J. Chen. 2006. Comparative observation of protective effects of earplug and barrel on auditory organs of guinea pigs exposed to experimental blast underpressure. *Chinese Journal of Traumatology* 9(4):242-245.

Lippa, S. M., N. J. Pastorek, J. F. Benge, and G. M. Thornton. 2010. Postconcussive symptoms after blast and nonblast-related mild traumatic brain injuries in Afghanistan and Iraq War veterans. *Journal of the International Neuropsychological Society* 16(5):856-866.

Mac Donald, C. L., A. M. Johnson, D. Cooper, E. C. Nelson, N. J. Werner, J. S. Shimony, A. Z. Snyder, M. E. Raichle, J. R. Witherow, R. Fang, S. F. Flaherty, and D. L. Brody. 2011. Detection of blast-related traumatic brain injury in U.S. military personnel. *New England Journal of Medicine* 364(22):2091-2100.

Magnuson, J., F. Leonessa, and G. S. F. Ling. 2012. Neuropathology of explosive blast traumatic brain injury. *Current Neurology and Neuroscience Reports* 12(5):570-579.

Magone, M. T., G. C. Cockerham, and S. Y. Shin. 2013. Visual dysfunction in combat related mild traumatic brain injury: A review. *US Ophthalmic Review* 6(1):48-51.

Markell, K. W., E. M. Renz, C. E. White, M. E. Albrecht, L. H. Blackbourne, M. S. Park, D. A. Barillo, K. K. Chung, R. A. Kozar, J. P. Minei, S. M. Cohn, D. N. Herndon, L. C. Cancio, J. B. Holcomb, and S. E. Wolf. 2009. Abdominal complications after severe burns. *Journal of the American College of Surgeons* 208(5):940-947; discussion 947-949.

Matthews, S., A. Simmons, and I. Strigo. 2011. The effects of loss versus alteration of consciousness on inhibition-related brain activity among individuals with a history of blast-related concussion. *Psychiatry Research* 191(1):76-79.

Matthews, S. C., A. D. Spadoni, J. B. Lohr, I. A. Strigo, and A. N. Simmons. 2012. Diffusion tensor imaging evidence of white matter disruption associated with loss versus alteration of consciousness in warfighters exposed to combat in Operations Enduring and Iraqi Freedom. *Psychiatry Research* 204(2-3):149-154.

Mayorga, M. A. 1997. The pathology of primary blast overpressure injury. *Toxicology* 121(1):17-28.

McEntire, B. J., and P. Whitely. 2005. Blunt Impact Performance Characteristics of the Advanced Combat Helmet and the Paratrooper and Infantry Personnel Armor System for Ground Troops Helmet. USAARL 2005-12 US Army Aeromedical Research Laboratory.

McKee, A. C., T. D. Stein, C. J. Nowinski, R. A. Stern, D. H. Daneshvar, V. E. Alvarez, H. S. Lee, G. Hall, S. M. Wojtowicz, C. M. Baugh, D. O. Riley, C. A. Kubilus, K. A. Cormier, M. A. Jacobs, B. R. Martin, C. R. Abraham, T. Ikezu, R. R. Reichard, B. L. Wolozin, A. E. Budson, L. E. Goldstein, N. W. Kowall, and R. C. Cantu. 2012. The spectrum of disease in chronic traumatic encephalopathy. *Brain* Jan;136(Pt 1):43-64.

McKibben, J. B., L. Ekselius, D. C. Girasek, N. F. Gould, C. Holzer, M. Rosenberg, S. Dissanaike, and A. C. Gielen. 2009. Epidemiology of burn injuries II: Psychiatric and behavioural perspectives. *International Review of Psychiatry* 21(6):512-521.

Mendez, M. F., E. M. Owens, E. E. Jimenez, D. Peppers, and E. A. Licht. 2013. Changes in personality after mild traumatic brain injury from primary blast vs. blunt forces. *Brain Injury* 27(1):10-18.

Mesquita-Guimaraes, J., F. Azevedo, and S. Aguiar. 1987. Silica granulomas secondary to the explosion of a land mine. *Cutis* 40(1):41-43.

Mody, R. M., M. Zapor, J. D. Hartzell, P. M. Robben, P. Waterman, R. Wood-Morris, R. Trotta, R. C. Andersen, and G. Wortmann. 2009. Infectious complications of damage control orthopedics in war trauma. *Journal of Trauma: Injury, Infection, & Critical Care* 67(4):758-761.

Morley, M. G., J. K. Nguyen, J. S. Heier, B. J. Shingleton, J. F. Pasternak, and K. S. Bower. 2010. Blast eye injuries: A review for first responders. *Disaster Medicine & Public Health Preparedness* 4(2):154-160.

Mossadegh, S., N. Tai, M. Midwinter, and P. Parker. 2012. Improvised explosive device related pelvi-perineal trauma: Anatomic injuries and surgical management. *Journal of Trauma and Acute Care Surgery* 73(2 Suppl 1):S24-S31.

Murray, C. K. 2008a. Epidemiology of infections associated with combat-related injuries in Iraq and Afghanistan. *Journal of Trauma: Injury, Infection, & Critical Care* 64(3 Suppl):S232-S238.

Murray, C. K. 2008b. Infectious disease complications of combat-related injuries. *Critical Care Medicine* 36(7 Suppl):S358-S364.

Murray, C. K., J. C. Reynolds, J. M. Schroeder, M. B. Harrison, O. M. Evans, and D. R. Hospenthal. 2005. Spectrum of care provided at an echelon II medical unit during Operation Iraqi Freedom. *Military Medicine* 170(6):516-520.

Murray, C. K., F. L. Loo, D. R. Hospenthal, L. C. Cancio, J. A. Jones, S. H. Kim, J. B. Holcomb, C. E. Wade, and S. E. Wolf. 2008. Incidence of systemic fungal infection and related mortality following severe burns. *Burns* 34(8):1108-1112.

Murray, C. K., H. C. Yun, M. E. Griffith, B. Thompson, H. K. Crouch, L. S. Monson, W. K. Aldous, K. Mende, and D. R. Hospenthal. 2009. Recovery of multidrug-resistant bacteria from combat personnel evacuated from Iraq and Afghanistan at a single military treatment facility. *Military Medicine* 174(6):598-604.

Murray, C. K., K. Wilkins, N. C. Molter, F. Li, L. Yu, M. A. Spott, B. Eastridge, L. H. Blackbourne, and D. R. Hospenthal. 2011. Infections complicating the care of combat casualties during Operations Iraqi Freedom and Enduring Freedom. *Journal of Trauma: Injury, Infection, & Critical Care* 71(1 Suppl):S62-S73.

NATO (North Atlantic Treaty Organization). 2004. *Test Methodologies for Personal Protective Equipment Against Anti-Personnel Mine Blast.* Research Technology Organization. http://ftp.rta.nato.int/public//PubFullText/RTO/TR/RTO-TR-HFM-089///TR-HFM-089-$$TOC.pdf (accessed November 13, 2013).

Needham, D. M., J. Davidson, H. Cohen, R. O. Hopkins, C. Weinert, H. Wunsch, C. Zawistowski, A. Bemis-Dougherty, S. C. Berney, O. J. Bienvenu, S. L. Brady, M. B. Brodsky, L. Denehy, D. Elliott, C. Flatley, A. L. Harabin, C. Jones, D. Louis, W. Meltzer, S. R. Muldoon, J. B. Palmer, C. Perme, M. Robinson, D. M. Schmidt, E. Scruth, G. R. Spill, C. P. Storey, M. Render, J. Votto, and M. A. Harvey. 2012. Improving long-term outcomes after discharge from intensive care unit: Report from a stakeholders' conference. *Critical Care Medicine* 40(2):502-509.

Nelson, E. R., V. W. Wong, P. H. Krebsbach, S. C. Wang, and B. Levi. 2012a. Heterotopic ossification following burn injury: The role of stem cells. *Journal of Burn Care & Research* 33(4):463-470.

Nelson, N. W., J. B. Hoelzle, B. M. Doane, K. A. McGuire, A. G. Ferrier-Auerbach, M. J. Charlesworth, G. J. Lamberty, M. A. Polusny, P. A. Arbisi, and S. R. Sponheim. 2012b. Neuropsychological outcomes of U.S. Veterans with report of remote blast-related concussion and current psychopathology. *Journal of the International Neuropsychological Society* 18(5):845-855.

Norin, J. A., D. C. Emanuel, and T. R. Letowski. 2011. Speech intelligibility and passive, level-dependent earplugs. *Ear Hear* 32(5):642-649.

NRC (National Research Council). 2012. *Testing of Body Armor Materials: Phase III.* Washington, DC: The National Academies Press.

Oertel, M., W. J. Boscardin, W. D. Obrist, T. C. Glenn, D. L. McArthur, T. Gravori, J. H. Lee, and N. A. Martin. 2005. Posttraumatic vasospasm: The epidemiology, severity, and time course of an underestimated phenomenon: A prospective study performed in 299 patients. *Journal of Neurosurgery* 103(5):812-824.

Okie, S. 2005. Traumatic brain injury in the war zone. *New England Journal of Medicine* 352(20):2043-2047.

Owens, B. D., J. F. Kragh, Jr., J. C. Wenke, J. Macaitis, C. E. Wade, and J. B. Holcomb. 2008. Combat wounds in Operation Iraqi Freedom and Operation Enduring Freedom. *Journal of Trauma: Injury, Infection, & Critical Care* 64(2):295-299.

Owers, C., J. L. Morgan, and J. P. Garner. 2011. Abdominal trauma in primary blast injury. *British Journal of Surgery* 98(2):168-179.

Ozer, O., I. Sari, V. Davutoglu, and C. Yildirim. 2009. Pericardial tamponade consequent to a dynamite explosion: Blast overpressure injury without penetrating trauma. *Texas Heart Institute Journal* 36(3):259-260.

Paolino, K. M., J. A. Henry, D. R. Hospenthal, G. W. Wortmann, and J. D. Hartzell. 2012. Invasive fungal infections following combat-related injury. *Military Medicine* 177(6):681-685.

Paquette, E. L. 2007. Genitourinary trauma at a combat support hospital during Operation Iraqi Freedom: The impact of body armor. *Journal of Urology* 177(6):2196-2199.

Peker, A. F., I. Yildirim, S. Bedir, F. Sumer, and M. Dayanc. 2002. Penile reconstruction with prosthesis and free skin graft in a patient with land mine blast injury. *Journal of Urology* 167(5):2133-2134.

Peleg, K., A. Liran, A. Tessone, A. Givon, A. Orenstein, and J. Haik. 2008. Do burns increase the severity of terror injuries? *Journal of Burn Care & Research* 29(6):887-892.

Penn-Barwell, J. G., C. A. Fries, I. D. Sargeant, P. M. Bennett, and K. Porter. 2012. Aggressive soft tissue infections and amputation in military trauma patients. *Journal of the Royal Naval Medical Service* 98(2):14-18.

Peral Gutierrez De Ceballos, J., F. Turegano Fuentes, D. Perez Diaz, M. Sanz Sanchez, C. Martin Llorente, and J. E. Guerrero Sanz. 2005. Casualties treated at the closest hospital in the Madrid, March 11, terrorist bombings. *Critical Care Medicine* 33(Suppl 1): S107-S112.

Peskind, E. R., E. C. Petrie, D. J. Cross, K. Pagulayan, K. McCraw, D. Hoff, K. Hart, C.-E. Yu, M. A. Raskind, D. G. Cook, and S. Minoshima. 2011. Cerebrocerebellar hypometabolism associated with repetitive blast exposure mild traumatic brain injury in 12 Iraq War veterans with persistent post-concussive symptoms. *Neuroimage* 54(Suppl 1):S76-S82.

Peterson, A. L., C. A. Luethcke, E. V. Borah, A. M. Borah, and S. Young-McCaughan. 2011. Assessment and treatment of combat-related PTSD in returning war veterans. *Journal of Clinical Psychology in Medical Settings* 18(2):164-175.

Phillips, Y. Y. 1986. Primary blast injuries. *Annals of Emergency Medicine* 15(12):1446-1450.

Phillips, Y. Y., and D. R. Richmond. 1991. Primary blast injury and basic research: A brief history. In *Conventional Warfare: Ballistic, Blast, and Burn Injuries*. Washington, DC: Office of the Surgeon General at TMM Publications. Pp. 221-240.

Phillips, Y. Y., T. G. Mundie, J. T. Yelverton, and D. R. Richmond. 1988. Cloth ballistic vest alters response to blast. *Journal of Trauma: Injury, Infection, & Critical Care* 28(1 Suppl):S149-S152.

Phillips, Y. Y., T. G. Mundie, R. Hoyt, and K. T. Dodd. 1989. Middle ear injury in animals exposed to complex blast waves inside an armored vehicle. *Annals of Otology, Rhinology, & Laryngology—Supplement* 140:17-22.

Polusny, M. A., S. M. Kehle, N. W. Nelson, C. R. Erbes, P. A. Arbisi, and P. Thuras. 2011. Longitudinal effects of mild traumatic brain injury and posttraumatic stress disorder comorbidity on postdeployment outcomes in National Guard soldiers deployed to Iraq. *Archives of General Psychiatry* 68(1):79-89.

Potter, B. K., T. C. Burns, A. P. Lacap, R. R. Granville, and D. A. Gajewski. 2007. Heterotopic ossification following traumatic and combat-related amputations: Prevalence, risk factors, and preliminary results of excision. *Journal of Bone & Joint Surgery—American Volume* 89(3):476-486.

Ragel, B. T., C. D. Allred, S. Brevard, R. T. Davis, and E. H. Frank. 2009. Fractures of the thoracolumbar spine sustained by soldiers in vehicles attacked by improvised explosive devices. *Spine* 34(22):2400-2405.

Ramasamy, A., A. M. Hill, S. D. Masouros, F. Gordon, J. C. Clasper, and A. M. J. Bull. 2011. Evaluating the effect of vehicle modification in reducing injuries from landmine blasts: An analysis of 2212 incidents and its application for humanitarian purposes. *Accident Analysis & Prevention* 43(5):1878-1886.

Ramasamy, A., S. Evans, J. M. Kendrew, and J. Cooper. 2012. The open blast pelvis: The significant burden of management. *Journal of Bone & Joint Surgery—British Volume* 94(6):829-835.

Resick, P. A., L. F. Williams, M. K. Suvak, C. M. Monson, and J. L. Gradus. 2012. Long-term outcomes of cognitive-behavioral treatments for posttraumatic stress disorder among female rape survivors. *Journal of Consulting and Clinical Psychology* 80(2):201-210.

Ressner, R. A., C. K. Murray, M. E. Griffith, M. S. Rasnake, D. R. Hospenthal, and S. E. Wolf. 2008. Outcomes of bacteremia in burn patients involved in combat operations overseas. *Journal of the American College of Surgeons* 206(3):439-444.

Ritenour, A. E., and T. W. Baskin. 2008. Primary blast injury: Update on diagnosis and treatment. *Critical Care Medicine* 36(7 Suppl):S311-S317.

Ritenour, A. E., L. H. Blackbourne, J. F. Kelly, D. F. McLaughlin, L. A. Pearse, J. B. Holcomb, and C. E. Wade. 2010. Incidence of primary blast injury in US military overseas contingency operations: A retrospective study. *Annals of Surgery* 251(6):1140-1144.

Rivera, J. C., J. C. Wenke, J. A. Buckwalter, J. R. Ficke, and A. E. Johnson. 2012. Posttraumatic osteoarthritis caused by battlefield injuries: The primary source of disability in warriors. *Journal of the American Academy of Orthopaedic Surgeons* 20(Suppl 1):S64-S69.

Riviere, S., V. Schwoebel, K. Lapierre-Duval, G. Warret, M. Saturnin, P. Avan, A. Job, and T. Lang. 2008. Hearing status after an industrial explosion: Experience of the AZF explosion, 21 September 2001, France. *International Archives of Occupational and Environmental Health* 81(4):409-414.

Rona, R. J., N. T. Fear, L. Hull, and S. Wessely. 2007. Women in novel occupational roles: Mental health trends in the UK armed forces. *International Journal of Epidemiology* 36(2):319-326.

Rona, R. J., M. Jones, N. T. Fear, L. Hull, D. Murphy, L. Machell, B. Coker, A. C. Iversen, N. Jones, A. S. David, N. Greenberg, M. Hotopf, and S. Wessely. 2012. Mild traumatic brain injury in UK military personnel returning from Afghanistan and Iraq: Cohort and cross-sectional analyses. *Journal of Head Trauma Rehabilitation* 27(1):33-44.

Ruff, R. L., S. S. Ruff, and X. F. Wang. 2008. Headaches among Operation Iraqi Freedom/Operation Enduring Freedom veterans with mild traumatic brain injury associated with exposures to explosions. *Journal of Rehabilitation Research and Development* 45(7):941-952.

Ruskin, A., and O. W. Beard. 1948. The Texas City disaster: Cardiovascular studies, with followup results. *Texas Reports on Biology and Medicine* 6(2):234-259.

Ruskin, A., O. W. Beard, and R. L. Schaffer. 1948. Blast hypertension: Elevated arterial pressures in the victims of the Texas City disaster. *American Journal of Medicine* 4(2):228-236.

Salinas, N. L., and J. A. Faulkner. 2010. Facial trauma in Operation Iraqi Freedom casualties: An outcomes study of patients treated from April 2006 through October 2006. *Journal of Craniofacial Surgery* 21(4):967-970.

Savolainen, S., and K. M. Lehtomaki. 1997. Impulse noise and acute acoustic trauma in Finnish conscripts. Number of shots fired and safe distances. *Scandinavian Audiology* 26(2):122-126.

Sayer, N. A. 2012. Traumatic brain injury and its neuropsychiatric sequelae in war veterans. *Annual Review of Medicine* 63:405-419.

Sayer, N. A., C. E. Chiros, B. Sigford, S. Scott, B. Clothier, T. Pickett, and H. L. Lew. 2008. Characteristics and rehabilitation outcomes among patients with blast and other injuries sustained during the Global War on Terror. *Archives of Physical Medicine & Rehabilitation* 89(1):163-170.

Scekic, M., D. Ignjatovic, M. Duknic, and P. Janjic. 1991. Secondary perforation of the colon in a patient with blast injury of the abdomen: Case report. *Vojnosanitetski Pregled* 48(6):562-563.

Scheibel, R. S., M. R. Newsome, M. Troyanskaya, X. Lin, J. L. Steinberg, M. Radaideh, and H. S. Levin. 2012. Altered brain activation in military personnel with one or more traumatic brain injuries following blast. *Journal of the International Neuropsychological Society* 18(1):89-100.

Scherer, M., H. Burrows, R. Pinto, and E. Somrack. 2007. Characterizing self-reported dizziness and otovestibular impairment among blast-injured traumatic amputees: A pilot study. *Military Medicine* 172(7):731-737.

Schneider, J. C., and H. D. Qu. 2011. Neurologic and musculoskeletal complications of burn injuries. *Physical Medicine in Rehabilitation Clinics of North America* 22(2):261-275.

Schnurr, P. P., C. A. Lunney, A. Sengupta, and L. C. Waelde. 2003. A descriptive analysis of PTSD chronicity in Vietnam Veterans. *Journal of Traumatic Stress* 16(6):545-553.

Schoenfeld, A. J., R. L. Newcomb, M. P. Pallis, J. A. Serrano, J. O. Bader, and B. R. Waterman. 2013. Characterization of spinal injuries sustained by American service members killed in Iraq and Afghanistan: A study of 2,089 instances of spine trauma. *Journal of Trauma & Acute Care Surgery* 74(4):1112-1118.

Schofield, C. M., C. K. Murray, E. E. Horvath, L. C. Cancio, S. H. Kim, S. E. Wolf, and D. R. Hospenthal. 2007. Correlation of culture with histopathology in fungal burn wound colonization and infection. *Burns* 33(3):341-346.

Schweickert, W. D., and J. Hall. 2007. ICU-acquired weakness. *Chest* 131(5):1541-1549.

Scott, B. A., J. R. Fletcher, M. W. Pulliam, and R. D. Harris. 1986. The Beirut terrorist bombing. *Neurosurgery* 18(1):107-110.

Serkin, F. B., D. W. Soderdahl, J. Hernandez, M. Patterson, L. Blackbourne, and C. E. Wade. 2010. Combat urologic trauma in US military overseas contingency operations. *Journal of Trauma: Injury, Infection, & Critical Care* 69(Suppl 1):S175-S178.

Shah, F. A., F. Pike, K. Alvarez, D. Angus, A. B. Newman, O. Lopez, J. Tate, V. Kapur, A. Wilsdon, J. A. Krishnan, N. Hansel, D. Au, M. Avdalovic, V. S. Fan, R. G. Barr, and S. Yende. 2013. Bidirectional relationship between cognitive function and pneumonia. *American Journal of Respiratory & Critical Care Medicine* 188(5):586-592.

Shariat, S., S. Mallonee, E. Kruger, K. Farmer, and C. North. 1999. A prospective study of long-term health outcomes among Oklahoma City bombing survivors. *Journal—Oklahoma State Medical Association* 92(4):178-186.

Sherwood, J. E., S. Fraser, D. M. Citron, H. Wexler, G. Blakely, K. Jobling, and S. Patrick. 2011. Multi-drug resistant *Bacteroides fragilis* recovered from blood and severe leg wounds caused by an improvised explosive device (IED) in Afghanistan. *Anaerobe* 17(4):152-155.

Shively, S. B., and D. P. Perl. 2012. Traumatic brain injury, shell shock, and posttraumatic stress disorder in the military—past, present, and future. *Journal of Head Trauma Rehabilitation* 27(3):234-239.

Silla, R. C., J. Fong, J. Wright, and F. Wood. 2006. Infection in acute burn wounds following the Bali bombings: A comparative prospective audit. *Burns* 32(2):139-144.

Simmons, J. W., C. E. White, J. D. Ritchie, M. O. Hardin, M. A. Dubick, and L. H. Blackbourne. 2011. Mechanism of injury affects acute coagulopathy of trauma in combat casualties. *Journal of Trauma: Injury, Infection, & Critical Care* 71(1 Suppl):S74-S77.

Smith, B., C. A. Wong, T. C. Smith, E. J. Boyko, and G. D. Gackstetter. 2009. Newly reported respiratory symptoms and conditions among military personnel deployed to Iraq and Afghanistan: A prospective population-based study. *American Journal of Epidemiology* 170(11):1433.

Sponheim, S. R., K. A. McGuire, S. S. Kang, N. D. Davenport, S. Aviyente, E. M. Bernat, and K. O. Lim. 2011. Evidence of disrupted functional connectivity in the brain after combat-related blast injury. *Neuroimage* 54(Suppl 1):S21-S29.

St. Onge, P., D. S. McIlwain, M. E. Hill, T. J. Walilko, and L. B. Bardolf. 2011. Marine Corps breacher training study: Auditory and vestibular findings. *US Army Medical Department Journal* 96-106.

Stein, N. R., M. A. Mills, K. Arditte, C. Mendoza, A. M. Borah, P. A. Resick, B. T. Litz, and S. S. Consortium. 2012. A scheme for categorizing traumatic military events. *Behavior Modification* 36(6):787-807.

Stevens, D. L., L. L. Laposky, P. McDonald, and I. Harris. 1988. Spontaneous gas gangrene at a site of remote injury: Localization due to circulating antitoxin. *Western Journal of Medicine* 148(2):204-205.

Stewart, W. F., A. Schechter, and B. K. Rasmussen. 1994. Migraine prevalence: A review of population-based studies. *Neurology* 44(6):17-23.

Svennevig, J. L., J. Vaage, A. Westheim, G. Hafsahl, and H. E. Refsum. 1989. Late sequelae of lung contusion. *Injury* 20(5):253-256.

Tanielian, T., and L. H. Jaycox. 2008. Invisible Wounds of War: Psychological and Cognitive Injuries, Their Consequences, and Services to Assist Recovery. Santa Monica, CA: RAND Corporation.

Tarmey, N. T., C. L. Park, O. J. Bartels, T. C. Konig, P. F. Mahoney, and A. J. Mellor. 2011. Outcomes following military traumatic cardiorespiratory arrest: A prospective observational study. *Resuscitation* 82(9):1194-1197.

Teasdale, G., and B. Jennett. 1974. Assessment of coma and impaired consciousness. A practical scale. *Lancet* 2(7872):81-84.

Teasdale, G., and B. Jennett. 1976. Assessment and prognosis of coma after head injury. *Acta Neurochirurgica* 34(1-4):45-55.

Theeler, B. J., and J. C. Erickson. 2009. Mild head trauma and chronic headaches in returning US soldiers. *Headache* 49(4):529-534.

Theeler, B. J., F. G. Flynn, and J. C. Erickson. 2010. Headaches after concussion in US soldiers returning from Iraq or Afghanistan. *Headache* 50(8):1262-1272.

Theeler, B. J., F. G. Flynn, and J. C. Erickson. 2012. Chronic daily headache in US Soldiers after concussion. *Headache* 52(5):732-738.

Thomas, R., J. G. McManus, A. Johnson, P. Mayer, C. Wade, and J. B. Holcomb. 2009. Ocular injury reduction from ocular protection use in current combat operations. *Journal of Trauma: Injury, Infection, & Critical Care* 66(4 Suppl):S99-S103.

Thompson, I. M., S. F. Flaherty, and A. F. Morey. 1998. Battlefield urologic injuries: The Gulf War experience. *Journal of the American College of Surgeons* 187(2):139-141.

Tintle, S. M., M. F. Baechler, G. P. Nanos, J. A. Forsberg, and B. K. Potter. 2012. Reoperations following combat-related upper-extremity amputations. *Journal of Bone & Joint Surgery—American Volume* 94(16):e1191-e1196.

Tribble, D. R., N. G. Conger, S. Fraser, T. D. Gleeson, K. Wilkins, T. Antonille, A. Weintrob, A. Ganesan, L. J. Gaskins, P. Li, G. Grandits, M. L. Landrum, D. R. Hospenthal, E. V. Millar, L. H. Blackbourne, J. R. Dunne, D. Craft, K. Mende, G. W. Wortmann, R. Herlihy, J. McDonald, and C. K. Murray. 2011. Infection-associated clinical outcomes in hospitalized medical evacuees after traumatic injury: Trauma infectious disease outcome study. *Journal of Trauma: Injury, Infection, & Critical Care* 71(1 Suppl):S33-S42.

Trudeau, D. L., J. Anderson, L. M. Hansen, D. N. Shagalov, J. Schmoller, S. Nugent, and S. Barton. 1998. Findings of mild traumatic brain injury in combat veterans with PTSD and a history of blast concussion. *Journal of Neuropsychiatry & Clinical Neurosciences* 10(3):308-313.

Tucker, K., and A. Lettin. 1975. The Tower of London bomb explosion. *British Medical Journal* 3(5978):287-290.

US Army. 2010. Operator Manual for Improved Outer Tactical Vest (IOTV) and Improved Outer Tactical Vest Gen II (IOTV GEN II) Part of the Interceptor Body Armor System. TM 10-8470-208-10 US Army.

VA (Department of Veterans Affairs). 2011. *Annual Benefits Report Fiscal Year 2011.* http://www.publichealth.va.gov/docs/epidemiology/healthcare-utilization-report-fy2013-qtr1.pdf (accessed November 13, 2013).

VA. 2013. *Analysis of VA Health Care Utilization Among Operation Enduring Freedom (OEF), Operation Iraqi Freedom (OIF), and Operation New Dawn (OND) Veterans.* Washington, DC: Department of Veterans Affairs. http://www.publichealth.va.gov/docs/epidemiology/healthcare-utilization-report-fy2013-qtr1.pdf (accessed November 20, 2013).

VA and DOD. 2009. *Clinical Practice Guideline: Management of Concussion/Mild Traumatic Brain Injury.* http://www.healthquality.va.gov/mtbi/concussion_mtbi_full_1_0.pdf (accessed November 20, 2013).

Vadivelu, S., R. S. Bell, B. Crandall, T. DeGraba, and R. A. Armonda. 2010. Delayed detection of carotid-cavernous fistulas associated with wartime blast-induced craniofacial trauma. *Neurosurgical Focus* 28(5):E6.

Valiyaveettil, M., Y. Alamneh, S. A. Miller, R. Hammamieh, Y. Wang, P. Arun, Y. Wei, S. Oguntayo, and M. P. Nambiar. 2012. Preliminary studies on differential expression of auditory functional genes in the brain after repeated blast exposures. *Journal of Rehabilitation Research & Development* 49(7):1153-1162.

Van Campen, L. E., J. M. Dennis, R. C. Hanlin, S. B. King, and A. M. Velderman. 1999a. One-year audiologic monitoring of individuals exposed to the 1995 Oklahoma City bombing. *Journal of the American Academy of Audiology* 10(5):231-247.

Van Campen, L. E., J. M. Dennis, S. B. King, R. C. Hanlin, and A. M. Velderman. 1999b. One-year vestibular and balance outcomes of Oklahoma City bombing survivors. *Journal of the American Academy of Audiology* 10(9):467-483.

Vanderploeg, R. D., H. G. Belanger, R. D. Horner, A. M. Spehar, G. Powell-Cope, S. L. Luther, and S. G. Scott. 2012. Health outcomes associated with military deployment: Mild traumatic brain injury, blast, trauma, and combat associations in the Florida National Guard. *Archives of Physical Medicine and Rehabilitation* 93(11):1887-1895.

Verfaellie, M., G. Lafleche, A. Spiro, 3rd, C. Tun, and K. Bousquet. 2013. Chronic postconcussion symptoms and functional outcomes in OEF/OIF veterans with self-report of blast exposure. *Journal of the International Neuropsychological Society* 19(1):1-10.

Vuckovic, I., A. Tucak, J. Gotovac, B. Karlovic, I. Matos, K. Grdovic, and M. Zelic. 1995. Croatian experience in the treatment of 629 urogenital war injuries. *Journal of Trauma: Injury, Infection, & Critical Care* 39(4):733-736.

Walker, W. C., S. D. McDonald, J. M. Ketchum, M. Nichols, and D. X. Cifu. 2013. Identification of transient altered consciousness induced by military-related blast exposure and its relation to postconcussion symptoms. *Journal of Head Trauma Rehabilitation* 28(1):68-76.

Walsh, R. M., J. P. Pracy, A. M. Huggon, and M. J. Gleeson. 1995. Bomb blast injuries to the ear: The London Bridge incident series. *Journal of Accident & Emergency Medicine* 12(3):194-198.

Wani, I., F. Q. Parray, T. Sheikh, R. A. Wani, A. Amin, I. Gul, and M. Nazir. 2009. Spectrum of abdominal organ injury in a primary blast type. *World Journal of Emergency Surgery* 4:46.

Warkentien, T., C. Rodriguez, B. Lloyd, J. Wells, A. Weintrob, J. R. Dunne, A. Ganesan, P. Li, W. Bradley, L. J. Gaskins, F. Seillier-Moiseiwitsch, C. K. Murray, E. V. Millar, B. Keenan, K. Paolino, M. Fleming, D. R. Hospenthal, G. W. Wortmann, M. L. Landrum, M. G. Kortepeter, and D. R. Tribble. 2012. Invasive mold infections following combat-related injuries. *Clinical Infectious Diseases* 55(11):1441-1449.

WHO (World Health Organization). 2010. *International Statistical Classification of Diseases and Related Health Problems.* 10th ed. http://apps.who.int/classifications/icd10/browse/2010/en#/F43.0 (accessed November 20, 2013).

Wiechman, S. A. 2011. Psychosocial recovery, pain, and itch after burn injuries. *Physical Medicine and Rehabilitation Clinics of North America* 22(2):327-345.

Wijekoon, C. J., K. H. Weerasekera, and A. K. Weerasinghe. 1995. Sarcoid-like granulomas of the skin seven years after bomb blast injury. *Ceylon Medical Journal* 40(3):126-127.

Wilk, J. E., R. K. Herrell, G. H. Wynn, L. A. Riviere, and C. W. Hoge. 2012. Mild traumatic brain injury (concussion), posttraumatic stress disorder, and depression in U.S. soldiers involved in combat deployments: Association with postdeployment symptoms. *Psychosomatic Medicine* 74(3):249-257.

Wilkinson, C. W., K. F. Pagulayan, E. C. Petrie, C. L. Mayer, E. A. Colasurdo, J. B. Shofer, K. L. Hart, D. Hoff, M. A. Tarabochia, and E. R. Peskind. 2012. High prevalence of chronic pituitary and target-organ hormone abnormalities after blast-related mild traumatic brain injury. *Frontiers in Neurology* 3:11.

Wisse, R. P., W. R. Bijlsma, and J. S. Stilma. 2010. Ocular firework trauma: A systematic review on incidence, severity, outcome and prevention. *British Journal of Ophthalmology* 94(12):1586-1591.

Wolf, D. G., I. Polacheck, C. Block, C. L. Sprung, M. Muggia-Sullam, Y. G. Wolf, A. Oppenheim-Eden, A. Rivkind, and M. Shapiro. 2000. High rate of candidemia in patients sustaining injuries in a bomb blast at a marketplace: A possible environmental source. *Clinical Infectious Diseases* 31(3):712-716.

Wolf, S. E., D. S. Kauvar, C. E. Wade, L. C. Cancio, E. P. Renz, E. E. Horvath, C. E. White, M. S. Park, S. Wanek, M. A. Albrecht, L. H. Blackbourne, D. J. Barillo, and J. B. Holcomb. 2006. Comparison between civilian burns and combat burns from Operation Iraqi Freedom and Operation Enduring Freedom. *Annals of Surgery* 243(6):786-792.

Wood, G. W., M. B. Panzer, J. K. Shridharani, K. A. Matthews, B. P. Capehart, B. S. Myers, and C. R. Bass. 2012. Attenuation of blast pressure behind ballistic protective vests. *Injury Prevention* 19(1):19-25.

Xydakis, M. S., G. S. Ling, L. P. Mulligan, C. H. Olsen, and W. C. Dorlac. 2012. Epidemiologic aspects of traumatic brain injury in acute combat casualties at a major military medical center: A cohort study. *Annals of Neurology* 72(5):673-681.

Yzermans, C. J., G. A. Donker, J. J. Kerssens, A. J. E. Dirkzwager, R. J. H. Soeteman, and P. M. H. ten Veen. 2005. Health problems of victims before and after disaster: A longitudinal study in general practice. *International Journal of Epidemiology* 34(4):820-826.

Zachar, M. R., C. Labella, C. P. Kittle, P. B. Baer, R. G. Hale, and R. K. Chan. 2013. Characterization of mandibular fractures incurred from battle injuries in Iraq and Afghanistan from 2001-2010. *Journal of Oral & Maxillofacial Surgery* 71(4):734-742.

Zachariah, J. R., A. L. Rao, R. Prabha, A. K. Gupta, M. K. Paul, and S. Lamba. 2012. Post burn pruritus: A review of current treatment options. *Burns* 38(5):621-629.

Zanni, G. R. 2012. Thermal burns and scalds: Clinical complications in the elderly. *The Consultant Pharmacist* 27(1):16-22.

# 5

# Recommendations

This chapter summarizes key gaps in the evidence base on exposure to blast and long-term health effects and offers recommendations for scientific study to fill the gaps. Recommendations aimed at improving dissemination of information on health effects after exposure to blast throughout the Department of Veterans Affairs (VA) and the Department of Defense (DOD) also are presented.

## RESEARCH RECOMMENDATIONS

Because of the inadequacy of evidence on long-term consequences of blast, the committee relied heavily on the literature to assess the evidence on acute effects and on its own collective medical expertise to draw conclusions regarding the plausibility of long-term consequences. Some long-term effects are obvious and well-documented consequences of acute injuries, but others will require additional study. Gaps in data collection begin while service members are on active duty and continue after they separate from the military and enter the VA health care system.

A fundamental feature of exposure to blast is that it can result in complex, multisystem injuries. Attention to the complexities has been lacking in many research studies. *Research on blast should emphasize multisystem injury patterns and seek to understand the clinical importance of cross-system interactions.*

Below are the committee's recommendations for research that is most likely to provide VA with knowledge that it can use to inform decisions on how to prevent blast injuries, how to diagnose them effectively, and how to manage, treat, and rehabilitate victims of battlefield traumas in the immediate aftermath of a blast and in the long term.

### Evaluating Current Approaches to Detecting Blast Injuries and Treating and Rehabilitating the Injured

Through the literature evaluation process summarized in Chapter 4, the committee identified several long-term health outcomes on which there was sufficient evidence of an association with blast exposure. VA can begin to improve the diagnosis of and treatment for blast injuries, particularly health outcomes for which there is sufficient evidence of an association with exposure to blast, namely:

- Sufficient evidence of a causal relationship between penetrating eye injuries resulting from exposure to blast and permanent blindness and visual impairment (visual acuity of 20/40 or worse).
- Sufficient evidence of a causal relationship between exposure to blast and some long-term effects on a genitourinary organ—such as hypogonadism, infertility, voiding dysfunction, and erectile dysfunction—associated with severe injury (defined as a complete structural and functional loss that cannot be reconstructed).
- Sufficient evidence of an association between exposure to blast and posttraumatic stress disorder (PTSD); the association may be related to direct exposure of blast or to indirect exposure, such as witnessing the aftermath of a blast or being part of a community that is affected by a blast.
- Sufficient evidence of an association between severe or moderate blast-related traumatic brain injury (TBI) and endocrine dysfunction (hypopituitarism and growth hormone deficiency).
- Sufficient evidence of an association between mild blast TBI and postconcussive symptoms and persistent headache.
- Sufficient evidence of an association between severe or moderate non-blast-related TBI and permanent neurologic disability, including cognitive dysfunction, unprovoked seizures, and headache; these associations are known outcomes from TBI studies that considered blast and non-blast mechanisms together, and it is plausible that severe or moderate blast-related TBI is similarly associated with permanent neurologic disability even though studies specifically addressing blast-related TBI are lacking.
- Sufficient evidence of an association between exposure to blast and long-term dermal effects, such as cutaneous granulomas.

Recommendation 5-1. The Department of Veterans Affairs should conduct a rigorous evaluation to determine whether current approaches for detecting, treating for, and rehabilitating after health outcomes of blast exposure are adequate.

Because exposure to blast is likely to lead to polytrauma that may affect many organ systems both acutely and in the long term, VA should assess its ability to coordinate care of blast survivors who have several health conditions. VA should assess the adequacy of current approaches to management of multiple chronic conditions, such as rehabilitation, and of its long-term followup care in treating blast survivors. For example, the agency should evaluate the extent to which Patient Aligned Care Teams (PACTs) provide adequate polytrauma care of patients who have been exposed to blast.

Current or newly developed approaches for rehabilitation should be evaluated with appropriately designed studies that include adequate control groups. The impact of rehabilitation services on long-term consequences of blast exposure should be assessed according to quality of life and measures of activity and participation, such as employment status, family relations, and independence in activities of daily living.

### Measuring Blast Exposure

A limitation of nearly all of the studies evaluated by the committee was inadequate information about the exposures to blast. Most of the studies used self-reported exposure data rather than objective measures. Obtaining accurate, objective measurement of exposure to blast is essential for understanding the mechanisms of injury caused by blast and for developing effective prevention and treatment strategies.

Recommendation 5-2. The Department of Defense should develop and deploy a system that measures essential components of blast and characteristics of the exposure environment, that records and stores the collected information, and that links individual blast-exposure databases with self-reported information and with demographic, medical, and operational data.

The system should measure components of primary, secondary, tertiary, quaternary, and quinary (radiation) blast. These components should include

- pressure—static, dynamic, and total;
- blast signature—impulse, primary peak, and refraction waves, intensity and duration of refraction waves;
- blast-wave frequency;

- impact and kinetic energy;
- acceleration;
- temperature;
- ionization;
- time stamp; and
- environmental factors, such as ground configuration (open field, confined space in a vehicle or building, and complexity), gas exhaust, and noise.

The components would be measured by sensors providing 360-degree coverage; by covering critical body regions (head, chest, and abdomen); and by using individual, helmet-mounted cameras. The sensors' and cameras' recordings would be triggered by blast.

The data would be temporarily stored in a small storage unit worn on the body. The storage unit would collect information from multiple sensors that are triggered by blast and would incorporate the information into one identifiable event. The unit would be capable of recording data on multiple events. After completion of the military task, the information in the individual storage units would be downloaded onto computers on a military base and stored in a large database. Much of the technology for the sensors and data-storage system has been developed (for example, helmet cameras are commonly worn by service members in the field), but research is needed to combine the various parts of the system into a wearable unit.

The body's physiologic status at the time of trauma may play a substantial role in injury outcome, so measuring hydration status, body-fat percentage, and heart-rate variability with sensors triggered by blast would provide valuable information.

The individual databases containing information about blast events should be linkable to other databases that include the following information:

- occurrence of loss of consciousness;
- subjective sensations, such as dizziness, "seeing stars," ringing in the ears, breathing difficulties, dry cough or irritation, photophobia, and blurred near vision;
- acute post-blast medical reports, such as reports from a buddy-aid, medics, the evacuation physician at the field-hospital, and potential transport to a Level III hospital;
- previous exposures—number, intensity, complexity, and time between exposures;
- previous deployments—number, duration of each, and interval between deployments;
- previous injuries—blast and non-blast;

- previous military traumatic events—number, type, and level of distress;
- age, sex, rank, military occupational specialty code, education, and length of service;
- family status, children, and socioeconomic status;
- detailed individual and family medical history;
- results of psychologic and physical tests; and
- results of military performance evaluations.

The committee recognizes that implementing a system with those characteristics will take time, although some of the components already have been developed and fielded (personal communication, I. Cernak, University of Alberta, August 8, 2013). Until the new system is available, the following questionnaires can be used to provide an operational definition of blast exposure: Quantification of Cumulative Blast Exposure (Peskind et al., 2011), Warrior Administered Retrospective Casualty Assessment Tool (Terrio et al., 2009), and Post-deployment Health Assessment Questions 10.a and 10.b (DOD, 2012). Clearly defining those scales' interrelationships and comparability and developing approaches to allow integration of findings from the various questionnaires should be given high priority to advance blast science. Although important, the use of self-report scales documenting exposure to blast will be subject to the usual inconsistencies that are inherent to these scales. Additionally, in cases of frontal lobe injury, the accuracy of the reports will be further diminished by known deficits in self-awareness that follow that type of injury.

A research consensus process could be applied to develop, validate, and promote the use of a self-report blast exposure scale for use in clinical and epidemiologic studies to be used prior to and in combination with deployment of blast detection technology. An important limitation of existing clinical and epidemiologic studies is the lack of validated measures of blast exposure that capture its unique, multifaceted characteristics. For many veterans, quantification of blast exposure is limited to retrospective self-report with some supplementary information from combat records. A consensus process to measure blast exposure and promoting its use is important to improve the strength of the evidence of the long-term effects of blast exposure.

## Biomarkers of Blast Injury

Identification of blast injuries in service members, particularly injuries that are not acutely severe and may go undetected for long periods, presents a major challenge in both clinical and research settings. The ability to define biomarkers of blast injury that could serve as surrogates for exposure would constitute a substantial advance in the study of long-term outcomes of exposure to blast. Biomarkers are an active area of scientific research; however, the committee recognizes that scientific consensus is lacking on the potential for blast-injury research using blood and other body fluids to identify biomarkers of sufficient sensitivity and specificity to provide clinically useful prognostic or diagnostic utility. The committee believes that biomarker research has the potential to advance the understanding of the biology of a wide range of complex diseases, including blast injury. Many of the available studies in this field focus on potential biomarkers associated with TBI. For example, as described in Chapter 4, blast TBI may confer distinctive neuroimaging patterns as measured by diffusion tensor imaging; however, the evidence is preliminary and insufficient to permit any firm conclusions to be drawn.

As described in Chapter 4, novel neuroimaging techniques can elucidate structural and functional abnormalities in neurologic circuits that are not apparent in routine magnetic resonance imaging. Data from studies of various neurodegenerative diseases have identified promising biomarkers, such as spinal fluid or blood levels of axon neurofilament proteins, that relate to late outcomes of injury (Gaiottino et al., 2013; Petzold, 2005; Shaw et al., 2005). Serum proteins have also shown promise as biomarkers for the diagnosis of non-blast mild TBI. For example, the combined use of serum S100B and apolipoprotein A-1 values increases classification accuracy for mild TBI over either marker used alone, and serum S100B alone is predictive of an abnormal head CT scan (Bazarian et al., 2013).

Other reports of the National Academies support the committee's view on the transformative potential of modern biomarker research for many complex conditions (IOM, 2008, 2013; NRC, 2011). The 2008 Institute of Medicine (IOM) report *Neuroscience Biomarkers and Biosignatures: Converging Technologies, Emerging Partnerships* discusses how studies of genomic and proteomic biomarkers have shown promise in the field of neuroscience generally (IOM, 2008). The 2013 IOM report *Genome-Based Diagnostics: Demonstrating Clinical Utility in Oncology* notes that several genomic predictive markers of cancer treatment efficacy and safety are in clinical use and more are undergoing testing (IOM, 2013). The 2011 National Research Council report *Toward Precision Medicine: Building a Knowledge Network for Biomedical Research and a New Taxonomy of Disease* discusses how the use of large data sets is a way to clarify new mechanisms, pathways, and heterogeneity of chronic diseases (NRC, 2011). Such large data sets will allow for the integration of cohorts of individuals with unexplained illness.

The committee believes that the use of biomarkers will be an important component for integrating genomic data with imaging data and clinical observation, and will move science in the blast-injury field forward.

Recommendation 5-3. The Department of Veterans Affairs should conduct epidemiologic and mechanistic studies to identify biomarkers of blast injury.

For prospective definition of biomarkers of the signature blast injury that could be applied in future assessments, the committee recommends two complementary prospective studies. In the first study, a small number of service members enrolled in the Breacher Training Course, which includes exposure to blast, would be studied in detail to measure and control for blast exposure objectively. In the second, a larger separate cohort of service members would be studied in detail before and after deployment to allow comparison of those who were exposed to blast with those who were not. Both studies would involve measuring subject-specific changes in organ-specific structure and function. In the second study, blast exposure would be determined on the basis of self-reports, and all subjects would undergo identical predeployment and postdeployment organ-specific functional assessment. The assessment would include neuropsychologic testing, imaging, and collection of serum, plasma, whole blood, and other fluids (for example, cerebrospinal fluid) to assess blast-related changes in protein, genome, and transcriptome concentration as biomarkers.

The committee recognizes that some service members may be unaware of their injuries from blast and recommends that biomarker signatures defined in the above studies be applied to groups returning from deployment (perhaps by using existing data sets) who have developed chronic unexplained health problems (for example, PTSD, addiction, diffuse pain, communication difficulties, and headache) to establish whether any relationships exist between these conditions and clinically inapparent blast exposures. In addition, service members who are relatively asymptomatic from the standpoint of organ-specific injuries can be studied. The committee recommends comparing a large cohort of returning service members who have a history of blast exposure with those who do not (that is, conducting a nested case-control study). The service members can be examined on the basis of the biomarker signatures for evidence of asymptomatic disease and then followed longitudinally to detect differences between the groups in the latent development of adverse effects of blast on which the current literature is uninformative, including some disorders that have not yet been associated with blast. Cases and controls will need to be well matched for demographic factors and for organ-specific premorbid conditions that are known to affect outcome. Postmortem pathologic correlates would be a natural extension of this longitudinal study.

### Improving Collaboration in Blast-Injury Research

The committee identified substantial gaps in much of the published research on blast injuries. The gaps include inadequately powered data sets, incomplete control populations, and poor study designs; an absence of combat-relevant expertise in blast on the research team; and a need to refine and advance preclinical models so that they are adequately predictive of long-term multisystem effects of blast injuries in humans. Greater collaboration within and among institutions will expand the expertise of research teams and help to fill those gaps, and this approach should be considered a strength and not a limitation with respect to VA funding priorities.

> Recommendation 5-4. To support innovation and improve the state of blast science, the Department of Veterans Affairs should develop opportunities for multidisciplinary research collaborations that cross institutional barriers between the Veterans Health Administration, the Department of Defense, and other institutions.

### Improving Designs of Blast-Injury Studies

Most of the studies evaluated by the committee were limited by various aspects of their design, as described in Chapter 2. To assist VA and other researchers in improving the design of future studies, the committee offers several recommendations. In addition to the recommendations, it is important that all future studies use a standardized definition of blast exposure once it has been developed.

> Recommendation 5-5. The Department of Veterans Affairs should conduct research on acute and long-term consequences of blast injury involving all service members and veterans, not just users of the Veterans Health Administration.

> Recommendation 5-6. The Department of Veterans Affairs should create a registry of blast-exposed (not only blast-injured) service members to serve as a foundation for long-term studies.

> Recommendation 5-7. The Department of Veterans Affairs should use existing military records to identify a cohort of service members who served in the Iraq and Afghanistan wars to enroll in a prospective study of the long-term effects of blast on health and rehabilitation. The cohort should not be limited to service members who are known to have been exposed to blast.

Recommendation 5-8. The Department of Veterans Affairs should identify and use as a resource existing longitudinal cohort studies of populations that include blast-exposed service members and veterans. This resource may include information from existing ancillary studies of these cohorts to improve the detection and measurement of adverse long-term health outcomes of blast exposure.

The existing studies include longitudinal studies that were conceptualized and designed to look at other aspects of early adult life. The advantage of such studies is that they have good prospective collection of key risk factors or outcomes of interest before military service and blast exposure. With additional supplementary data collection, the studies' cohorts may provide important opportunities to answer specific questions about long-term health effects from exposure to blast, including the multisystem response to blast (for example, the complex relationship between TBI and PTSD). Illustrative examples include the National Longitudinal Study of Adolescent Health (2013), the Strong Star cohort (STRONG STAR, 2013), the Canadian Resilience Enhancement in Military Population longitudinal prospective study (Cernak, 2013), and selected Kaiser Permanente longitudinal studies (Kaiser Permanente, 2013).

Recommendation 5-9. The Department of Veterans Affairs should create a database linking Department of Defense records (particularly records that identify blast-injured service members) to records in the Veterans Health Administration, active-duty military treatment facilities, and TRICARE (the Department of Defense health care program) to facilitate identification of long-term health care needs after blast injury.

Recommendation 5-10. The Department of Veterans Affairs should conduct case-control studies of select adverse outcomes to test for the potential contribution of blast to them.

The case-control studies will be of particular value in incorporating biomarkers or other biologic signatures of blast that can be assessed retrospectively. The study design also will help to characterize clinically inapparent acute blast injuries.

## Identifying Predictors of Risk of Blast Injury

Screening tests on entry into the military (not only before deployment) should be helpful in gathering information on predictors of increased risk of blast injury. Before enlistment in the US military, applicants are required to undergo a physical examination, which includes height and weight measurements, hearing and visual examinations, urine and blood tests, muscle-group and joint maneuvers, drug and alcohol tests, a pregnancy test for women, and medical-history evaluation based on medical records or self-reported information (DOD, 2011). Specialized tests also may be required (for example, enlistees who are suspected of having epilepsy undergo a neurologic examination) (US Army, 2011). Having any of a number of pre-existing health conditions may exclude a person from serving (for example, see the Army's Standards of Medical Fitness; US Army, 2011).

**Recommendation 5-11. The Department of Defense should determine whether existing screening tests administered during the physical examination conducted on enlistment can be used to measure susceptibility to blast injury, and if additional screening tests might be helpful in determining whether a service member has an increased susceptibility to blast injury.**

In making the determination, the following questions should be considered:

- Do some biologic markers predict an increased risk of long-term effects of blast injury?
  o Which markers should be included? Some examples are genomic markers of susceptibility, baseline brain function and anatomy, baseline hearing function, and risk of alcohol and substance abuse.
  o What tests can be conducted? Some examples are auditory testing and ocular evaluation (contrast sensitivity, reading speed, and dry-eye quantification).
  o What investigative tests need to be developed? Some examples are DNA collection (such as genome-wide association studies and microarray assays) and brain imaging.
- Do some clinical characteristics predict an increased risk of the long-term effects of blast injury? The characteristics might include demographic variables, medical history, psychologic and psychiatric history or symptoms, resilience, and social and family support.
  o Which clinical characteristics should be included? Some examples are early-life trauma, family history of psychopathologic conditions, social support, and perceived life threat during traumatic events.
  o What questionnaires should be given? Some examples are the Early Traumatic Inventory Short Form and the Adverse Childhood Experiences Form, comprehensive medical history, family history questionnaire, and social support questionnaire.
  o What investigative tests need to be developed?

## DISSEMINATION OF INFORMATION ABOUT BLAST INJURIES

As part of its charge, the committee was asked to offer recommendations for disseminating information about the health effects of blast exposure throughout VA for the purpose of improving care and benefits provided to veterans. This section briefly discusses relevant pieces of VA's educational and communications infrastructure that could be used for that purpose, with recommendations of ways to build on the existing infrastructure to improve the dissemination of information about the health effects of blast injuries.

VA has in place several mechanisms for disseminating information to its clinicians and other health care team members, and the committee believes that the existing infrastructure can be used as the foundation for educating caregivers and others about health effects of blast exposure. It is important for VA health care teams to consider exposure to blast as a possible cause of a veteran's health problems, and this is particularly true for veterans of the Iraq and Afghanistan wars. Proper diagnosis of health problems caused by exposure to blast will probably also lead to more effective treatment and equitable allocation of benefits.

VA has several clinical practice guidelines (CPGs) and other documents related to blast injuries. The Blasts and Explosions VA DOD General Guidance Pocket Guide (2004) provides guidance for clinicians on how to provide treatment in the immediate aftermath of an explosion. It also describes the types of injuries that are often associated with explosions. In addition, VA has developed CPGs for postdeployment health conditions, such as TBI and PTSD (VA and DOD, 2001, 2009, 2010). VA has published its method for disseminating and implementing its CPGs in Veterans Health Administration medical facilities (Nicholas et al., 2001; VA, undated). The method is summarized in Box 5-1.

VA clinicians are given military health-history pocket cards that include guidance on questions to ask veterans (VA, 2013a). Although some of the questions that are currently asked may lead a veteran to inform a clinician that he or she was exposed to blast (for example, "Did you see combat, enemy fire, or casualties?"), none of the questions mention blast specifically.

VA's Polytrauma and Blast-Related Injuries Quality Enhancement Research Initiative (PT-BRI QUERI) focuses on conducting research to improve health outcomes in veterans who have experienced TBI. Although other types of blast-related injuries—including auditory, ocular, respiratory, gastrointestinal, and renal injuries—are within its scope, they are not being investigated as far as the committee could determine (VA, 2013c). The PT-BRI QUERI works with VA's Physical Medicine and Rehabilitation Program Office and disseminates its findings through the VA health care system via such groups as the VHA Screening Coordination Workgroup, the VA National Polytrauma Pain Subcommittee, the VHA Tele-rehabilitation

---

**BOX 5-1**
**Methods for Disseminating and Implementing Clinical Practice**
**Guidelines in the Veterans Health Administration**

**Implementation**
- Dedicate the necessary resources (for example, staff) to make the necessary changes happen. Leadership support, local ownership, and teamwork all are essential for successful implementation of guidelines.
- Assess how current clinical practices compare to what is recommended in the guideline.
- Develop an implementation action plan to close the gaps between current clinical practice and the guideline.
- Test the implementation action plan in the clinical environment.

**Monitoring and Assessing the Implementation Efforts**
- Choose appropriate measures.
- Collect data.
- Interpret the results.
- Make changes as needed.

**Adoption**
- This final step in the implementation process is made by the leadership of the Veterans Health Administration.

SOURCE: VA, undated.

---

Field Work Group, the Polytrauma Rehabilitation Center Family Care Collaborative, the DOD–VA Family Transition Task Force, the National Center for PTSD, the DOD Amputation Patient Care Program, and the Defense and Veterans Brain Injury Center.

VA's Simulation Learning, Education and Research Network (SimLEARN) provides continuing education curricula and best practices on a variety of health care issues (VA, 2012). Local VA medical centers also offer training courses. However, none of the curricula offered at the national or local levels appears to address health effects specifically of exposure to blasts.

VA's National Center for PTSD offers a number of educational materials and other products for clinicians (VA, 2013b). Examples include continuing education courses for both VA and non-VA employees, information on how to assess PTSD, and practice recommendations for treating veterans who have PTSD and comorbid conditions.

Multiple other opportunities for dissemination of information to health care team members about blast injuries exist in the VA health care system. For example, VA has been moving to the medical home model called PACTs, and each veteran entering the VA system is assigned to a PACT (Reisinger et al., 2012). Because of the multidisciplinary, team-based approach to providing medical care, PACTs are an ideal mechanism for increasing awareness about health effects of blast exposures. Additional mechanisms include the use of clinical champions to serve as internal resources for clinicians, and learning (peer) networks to facilitate sharing of information and skills related to managing health effects of blast exposures.

> Recommendation 5-12. The Department of Veterans Affairs (VA) should build on its existing educational and communication infrastructure to educate its clinicians and other health care team members further about the health effects of blast exposure. Specific actions should be taken to
>
> - Develop clinical practice guidelines (CPGs) for blast-related injuries other than traumatic brain injury (TBI) and posttraumatic stress disorder (PTSD). The CPGs should be developed in collaboration with the Department of Defense and ideally would be used by both departments.
> - Expand the focus of the Polytrauma and Blast-Related Injuries Quality Enhancement Research Initiative to include injuries other than TBI and PTSD. Blast injuries and rehabilitation after them should be viewed through a wide clinical lens.
> - Offer continuing education credit courses on blast injury through the Simulation Learning, Education and Research Network and other relevant educational forums.
> - Convene periodic state-of-the-science conferences (for example, every 2 or 3 years) on the health effects of blast injuries. Such conferences would be convened ideally in collaboration with the Department of Defense, and possibly with selected professional associations, and the conference proceedings would be published (for example, in special issues or supplements of professional journals).
> - Establish a blast-injury literature clearinghouse or information repository that could be used as a resource for clinicians and researchers. It should be a joint effort of the VA and the Department of Defense.

- Use such mechanisms as the patient-aligned care teams, clinical champions, and learning networks to educate VA health care teams about the health effects of blast exposure.
- Encourage clinicians to ask veterans specifically about exposure to blasts. Develop standard screening questions specific to veterans' exposures to blast for integration into the VA electronic health record and as part of veterans' military histories. The screening questions should be listed on the military health-history pocket card.

## REFERENCES

Bazarian, J. J., B. J. Blyth, H. He, S. Mookeries, C. Jones, K Kiechle, R. Moynihan, S. M. Wojcik, W. D. Grant, L. M. Secreti, W. Triner, R. Moscati, A. Leinhart, G. L. Ellis, and J. Khan. 2013. Classification accuracy of serum apo A-I and S100B for the diagnosis of mild traumatic brain injury and prediction of abnormal initial head computed tomography scan. *Journal of Neurotrauma* 30(20):1747-1754.

Cernak, I. 2013. *Resilience Enhancement in Military Populations Through Multiple Health Status Assessments (REIM)*. https://rehabmed2.sitecore.ualberta.ca/Research/CFChair2/Resilience%20Enhancement%20in%20Military.aspx (accessed September 9, 2013).

DOD (Department of Defense). 2011. *Personnel Procurement: Military Entrance Processing Station (MEPS)*. http://www.apd.army.mil/pdffiles/r601_270.pdf (accessed September 9, 2013).

DOD. 2012. *DD Form 2796: Post Deployment Health Assessment*. http://www.dtic.mil/whs/directives/infomgt/forms/eforms/dd2796.pdf (accessed December 19, 2013).

Gaiottino, J., N. Norgren, R. Dobson, J. Topping, A. Nissim, A. Malaspina, J. P. Bestwick, A. U. Monsch, A. Regeniter, R. L. Lindberg, L. Kappos, D. Leppert, A. Petzold, G. Giocannoni, and J. Kuhle. 2013. Increased neurofilament light chain blood levels in neurodegenerative neurological diseases. *PLoS ONE* 8(9):e75091.

IOM (Institute of Medicine). 2008. *Neuroscience Biomarkers and Biosignatures: Converging Technologies, Emerging Partnerships: Workshop Summary*. Washington, DC: The National Academies Press.

IOM. 2013. *Genome-Based Diagnostics: Demonstrating Clinical Utility in Oncology: Workshop Summary*. Washington, DC: The National Academies Press.

Kaiser Permanente. 2013. *Current Research Studies*. http://www.dor.kaiser.org/external/DORExternal/research/studies.aspx (accessed August 26, 2013).

The National Longitudinal Study of Adolescent Health. 2013. *Add Health*. http://www.cpc.unc.edu/projects/addhealth (accessed August 26, 2013).

Nicholas, W., D. O. Farley, M. E. Vaiana, and S. Cretin. 2001. *Putting Practice Guidelines to Work in the Department of Defense Medical System*. Santa Monica, CA: RAND Corporation. http://www.rand.org/content/dam/rand/pubs/monograph_reports/2007/MR1267.pdf (accessed August 26, 2013).

NRC (National Research Council). 2011. *Toward Precision Medicine: Building a Knowledge Network for Biomedical Research and a New Taxonomy of Disease*. Washington, DC: The National Academies Press.

Peskind, E. R., E. C. Petrie, D. J. Cross, K. Pagulayan, K. McCraw, D. Hoff, K. Hart, C.-E. Yu, M. A. Raskind, D. G. Cook, and S. Minoshima. 2011. Cerebrocerebellar hypometabolism associated with repetitive blast exposure mild traumatic brain injury in 12 Iraq War veterans with persistent post-concussive symptoms. *Neuroimage* 54(Suppl 1):S76-S82.

Petzold, A. 2005. Neurofilament phosphoforms: Surrogate markers for axonal injury, degeneration and loss. *Journal of the Neurological Sciences* 233(1-2):183-198.

Reisinger, H. S., S. C. Hunt, A. L. Burgo-Black, and M. A. Agarwal. 2012. A population approach to mitigating the long-term health effects of combat deployments. *Preventing Chronic Disease* 9:E54.

Shaw, G., C. Yang, R. Ellis, K. Anderson, J. Parker Mickle, S. Scheff, B. Pike, D. K. Anderson, D. R. Howland. 2005. Hyperphosphorylated neurofilament NF-H is a serum biomarker of axonal injury. *Biochemical and Biophysical Research Communications* 336(4):1268-1277.

STRONG STAR (South Texas Research Organization Network Guiding Studies on Trauma and Resilience). 2013. *Strong Star Research Projects: Finding the Best Ways to Prevent and Treat Combat-Related PTSD.* http://delta.uthscsa.edu/strongstar/research.asp (accessed August 26, 2013).

Terrio, H., L. A. Brenner, B. J. Ivins, J. M. Cho, K. Helmick, K. Schwab, K. Scally, R. Bretthauer, and D. Warden. 2009. Traumatic brain injury screening: Preliminary findings in a US Army brigade combat team. *Journal of Head Trauma Rehabilitation* 24(1):14-23.

US Army. 2011. *Standards of Medical Fitness.* Army Regulation 40-501. Department of Defense. http://www.apd.army.mil/pdffiles/r40_501.pdf (accessed August 26, 2013).

VA (Department of Veterans Affairs). 2012. *SimLEARN: National Curricula and Training.* http://www.simlearn.va.gov/SIMLEARN/Curricula_SimLEARN.asp (accessed 4/12/2013).

VA. 2013a. *Military Health History Pocket Card for Clinicians.* http://www.va.gov/oaa/pocketcard (accessed April 12, 2013).

VA. 2013b. *National Center for Posttraumatic Stress Disorder.* http://www.ptsd.va.gov/index.asp (accessed April 12, 2013).

VA. 2013c. *Polytrauma and Blast-Related Injuries Quality Enhancement Research Initiative.* http://www.queri.research.va.gov/ptbri (accessed April 12, 2013).

VA. Undated. *Putting Clinical Practice Guidelines to Work in VHA.* http://www.healthquality.va.gov/VA_Manual.pdf (accessed December 19, 2013).

VA and DOD. 2001. *Clinical Practice Guideline for Post-Deployment Health Evaluation and Management, Version 1.2.* http://www.healthquality.va.gov/pdh/PDH_cpg.pdf (accessed December 19, 2013).

VA and DOD. 2004. *Blasts and Explosions VA/DOD General Guidance Pocket Guide.* Washington, DC: Employee Education System for the Office of Public Health and Environmental Hazards and Patient Care Services of the Department of Veterans Affairs. http://www.oqp.med.va.gov/cpg/BCR/BCR_Base.htm (accessed December 19, 2013).

VA and DOD. 2009. *Clinical Practice Guideline: Management of Concussion/Mild Traumatic Brain Injury.* http://www.healthquality.va.gov/mtbi/concussion_mtbi_full_1_0.pdf (accessed December 19, 2013).

VA and DOD. 2010. *Clinical Practice Guideline for Management of Post-Traumatic Stress.* http://www.healthquality.va.gov/ptsd/PTSD-FULL-2010a.pdf (accessed December 19, 2013).

# Appendix

# Committee Biographic Information

**Stephen L. Hauser, MD** (*Chair*), is the Robert A. Fishman Distinguished Professor and chair of the Department of Neurology of the University of California, San Francisco (UCSF). Dr. Hauser is a graduate of the Massachusetts Institute of Technology (Phi Beta Kappa) and the Harvard Medical School (magna cum laude). He trained in internal medicine at the New York Hospital–Cornell Medical Center, in neurology at the Massachusetts General Hospital, and in immunology at the Harvard Medical School and the Institute Pasteur in Paris, France, and he was a faculty member of the Harvard Medical School before moving to UCSF in 1992. Dr. Hauser is a neuroimmunologist, and his research has advanced the understanding of the genetic basis and immune mechanisms and treatment for multiple sclerosis. He is a fellow of the American Academy of Arts and Sciences and of the American Academy of Physicians and is a member of the Institute of Medicine (IOM) of the National Academies. Dr. Hauser has served on several IOM committees and served as the chair of the Committee on Gulf War and Health: Health Effects of Serving in the Gulf War, Update 2009. He is an editor of the textbook *Harrison's Principles of Internal Medicine*, and editor-in-chief of *Annals of Neurology*. He has served as president of the American Neurological Association and president of the medical staff at UCSF. He also serves on several scientific advisory boards for nonprofit organizations. Dr. Hauser has received numerous awards and honors for his work, including the Jacob Javits Neuroscience Investigator Award and the 2008 John Dystel Prize for Multiple Sclerosis Research. In April, 2010, Dr. Hauser was appointed by President Obama to the Presidential Commission for the Study of Bioethical Issues, which is charged with advising the president on issues that may emerge from advances in biomedicine and related fields of science and technology.

**Jeffrey J. Bazarian, MD, MPH,** is associate professor of emergency medicine, neurology, and neurosurgery at the Center for Neural Development and Disease of the University of Rochester Medical Center. He graduated from Brown University and from the University of Rochester School of Medicine. He completed his residency training in internal medicine and has a master's degree in public health. Dr. Bazarian was one of the first emergency physicians to receive a 5-year Career Development Award from the National Institute of Neurological Disorders and Stroke. The focus of his research was traumatic brain injury (TBI) epidemiology and outcomes. Dr. Bazarian's research interest has recently shifted to finding better ways to diagnose TBI, especially concussion. He assembled a diverse group of researchers in the university to address the problem and created a translational research team. Those efforts earned him an R01 award in 2007 from the National Institute of Child Health and Human Development to develop a blood test for brain injury; he was one of only a handful of emergency physicians to receive such a grant. Dr. Bazarian has served on several TBI-related task forces and panels for the Centers for Disease Control and Prevention, the National Institutes of Health, and the National Science Foundation. He is currently serving on an Institute of Medicine committee that is examining readjustment needs in returning Iraq and Afghanistan active-duty military personnel, veterans, family members, and affected communities.

**Ibolja Cernak, MD, PhD, ME, MHS,** is the first chair of military and veterans' clinical rehabilitation in the University of Alberta, Canada. Dr. Cernak most recently was the medical director in the Biomedical Business Area of the Applied Physics Laboratory of Johns Hopkins University. Previously, she served on the battlefield as a first responder and conducted controlled clinical research to characterize complex neuroendocrine, neurologic, biochemical, and metabolic responses to blast exposure within the earliest posttraumatic period (0–5 minutes after trauma). Her research interests are in mechanisms of neuronal cell death and related neurologic deficits induced by traumatic brain injury, blunt head trauma, and war-induced (explosion-induced) blast neurotrauma. Dr. Cernak received her MD from the Medical School of the University of Belgrade, Yugoslavia; her MS in biomedical engineering from the Center of Multidisciplinary Studies of the University of Belgrade; her PhD in pathophysiology and neuroscience from the Military Medical Academy of the University of Belgrade; and her MS in homeland security in public health preparedness from the Pennsylvania State University. She has served on previous Institute of Medicine committees, including the Committee on Gulf War and Health: Brain Injury in Veterans and Long-Term Health Outcomes and the Committee on Readjustment Needs of Military Personnel, Veterans, and Their Families.

**Lin Chang, MD,** is a professor of medicine in the Department of Medicine, Division of Digestive Diseases, and the co-director of the Gail and Gerald Oppenheimer Center for Neurobiology of Stress of the David Geffen School of Medicine of University of California, Los Angeles. Dr. Chang's clinical expertise is in functional gastrointestinal disorders, which include irritable-bowel syndrome (IBS), chronic constipation, and functional dyspepsia. Her research focuses on the pathophysiology and health outcomes of IBS related to stress; sex differences, neuroendocrine alterations, and comorbidity with fibromyalgia; and treatment for IBS. She is a funded National Institutes of Health investigator studying the central and peripheral mechanisms that underlie IBS. She is the recipient of the Janssen Award in Gastroenterology for Basic or Clinical Research and the American Gastroenterological Association (AGA) Distinguished Clinician Award. Dr. Chang is the author of more than 80 original research articles, 50 review articles, and 19 book chapters on her specialty interests. She is a fellow of the AGA and the American College of Gastroenterology and a member of the Society for Neuroscience. She is also a member of the Rome Foundation Board of Directors. Dr. Chang is the president of the American Neurogastroenterology and Motility Society. She served on the Food and Drug Administration Gastrointestinal Drugs Advisory Committee from 2005 to 2010 and has also chaired the committee.

**Kimberly Cockerham, MD, FACS,** is a board-certified ophthalmologist in private practice in the Central Valley and Silicon Valley of California (Cupertino, Los Altos, Manteca, and Stockton). She is an adjunct clinical associate professor in the Department of Ophthalmology of Stanford University School of Medicine. Her professional affiliations include the American Academy of Ophthalmology, the North American Neuro-Ophthalmology Society, and the American Society of Ophthalmic Plastic and Reconstructive Surgery. Her past research work includes a Department of Defense grant for a reanimation of damaged nerve-muscle complexes administered through Palo Alto Institute for Research and Education at the Palo Alto Veterans Affairs (VA) Medical Center and a VA polytrauma study that investigated the effects of blast injuries on veterans of the Afghanistan and Iraq wars. Dr. Cockerham graduated with cum laude honors from the University of California San Diego. While serving for 15 years as an officer in the US Army, she obtained her MD from George Washington University Medical School and completed her internship in general surgery, her residency in ophthalmology, and two fellowships in neuro-ophthalmology and oculoplastics and orbital disease. In her final 5 years of military service, she was the director of oculoplastics and orbital surgery and reconstruction at Walter Reed Army Medical Center.

**Karen J. Cruickshanks, PhD,** is a professor of ophthalmology and visual sciences and population health sciences at the University of Wisconsin School of Medicine and Public Health. She completed her PhD in epidemiology at the University of Pittsburgh Graduate School of Public Health. Her research focuses on the epidemiology of age-related sensory disorders, cognitive impairment, and diabetes and its complications. The Epidemiology of Hearing Loss Study and the Beaver Dam Offspring Study are funded by the National Institute on Aging to study hearing, olfactory, and cognitive impairments in two population-based cohorts. Her professional affiliations include the Institute on Aging at the University of Wisconsin, the Society for Epidemiologic Research, the Association for Research in Vision and Ophthalmology, the American Epidemiological Society, the American Auditory Society, the Association for Chemoreception Sciences, and the American Heart Association. She has served on previous Institute of Medicine committees, including the Committee on Assessment of Noise-Induced Hearing Loss in the Military Service from WWII to the Present and the Committee to Review the National Institute for Occupational Safety and Health Hearing Loss Research Program.

**Francesca Dominici, PhD,** is a professor in the Department of Biostatistics of the Harvard School of Public Health and the associate dean of information technology. Dr. Dominici's research has focused on the interface between the methodologic development of hierarchic models and their applications to multilevel data. She has extensive experience in the development of statistical methods and their applications to clinical trials, toxicology, biology, and environmental epidemiology. She is a member of numerous professional societies, including the American Statistical Association, the International Biometric Society, and the International Society for Environmental Epidemiology. She is the senior editor of Chapman & Hall/ CRC Texts in Statistical Science series, and associate editor of the *Journal of the Royal Statistical Society*. Dr. Dominici has served on a number of National Academies committees, including the Committee on Gulf War and Health: Review of the Medical Literature Relative to Gulf War Veterans' Health; the Committee to Assess Potential Health Effects from Exposures to PAVE PAWS Low-Level Phased Array Radiofrequency Energy; and the Committee on the Utility of Proximity-Based Herbicide Exposure Assessment in Epidemiologic Studies of Vietnam Veterans. Dr. Dominici received her PhD in statistics from the University of Padua, Italy.

**Judy R. Dubno, PhD,** is a professor and director of research in the Department of Otolaryngology–Head and Neck Surgery of the Medical University of South Carolina in Charleston. Her research focuses on auditory perception, sensorineural hearing loss, and speech recognition. Dr. Dubno earned a PhD in speech and hearing science from the City University of New York Graduate Center and completed a postdoctoral fellowship at the University of California, Los Angeles, School of Medicine. Dr. Dubno's research on auditory-system function has improved the understanding of the encoding of auditory information in simple sounds and speech, and how those abilities change in adverse listening conditions and with training, age, and hearing loss. Dr. Dubno sits on editorial boards, national scientific boards, and National Institutes of Health (NIH) review panels. In addition to committee service in national scientific societies, she has served as president of the Association for Research in Otolaryngology, as a member of the NIH's National Institute on Deafness and Other Communication Disorders Advisory Council, and as vice president and president-elect of the Acoustical Society of America. She has served on previous Institute of Medicine committees, including the Committee on Noise-Induced Hearing Loss and Tinnitus Associated with Military Service from World War II to the Present and the Committee to Review the National Institute for Occupational Safety and Health Hearing Loss Research Program.

**Theodore J. Iwashyna, MD, PhD,** is an associate professor of internal medicine in the Division of Pulmonary and Critical Care Medicine of the University of Michigan. He is also a faculty associate of the Survey Research Center of the Institute for Social Research and a research scientist in the VA (Department of Veterans Affairs) Center for Clinical Management Research in Ann Arbor. His clinical interests are in the organization and outcomes of care for the critically ill; in particular, a major focus of his recent work has been understanding the causal links between severe sepsis and disability and cognitive impairment. Dr. Iwashyna is a member of several professional societies, including the American Thoracic Society and the Society of Critical Care Medicine. He received his AB from Princeton University in molecular biology, his MD from the Pritzker School of Medicine of the University of Chicago, and his PhD from the Harris School of Public Policy of the University of Chicago. He is board certified in internal medicine, pulmonary medicine, and critical care. He has grants from the National Heart, Lung, and Blood Institute, the VA Health Services Research and Development Service, and the Society of Critical Care Medicine.

**S. Claiborne Johnston, MD, PhD,** is a professor of neurology and epidemiology, associate vice chancellor of research, and director of the University of California, San Francisco (UCSF) Clinical and Translational Science

Institute. He received his undergraduate education at Amherst College and completed medical school at Harvard University. He received a PhD in epidemiology from the University of California, Berkeley. He completed his residency in neurology at UCSF, where he later trained in vascular neurology. Dr. Johnston is the author of more than 200 publications in scientific journals and has won several national awards for his research and teaching. He has led several large cohort studies of cerebrovascular disease and three multicenter randomized trials. He studies stroke treatment and prevention using the tools of computer science and epidemiology. Dr. Johnston is the executive vice editor of the Annals of Neurology and served on the editorial boards of several other journals. He has been honored with the American Academy of Neurology's Pessin Prize for Stroke Leadership and the American Stroke Association's Siekert New Investigator Award. He was a member of the California Health Disease and Stroke Prevention Advisory Council, which advises the Department of Health Services, and codirector of prevention education programs for the National Stroke Association.

S. Andrew Josephson, MD, is a neurologist who specializes in neurovascular and neurologic disorders. He is the director of the University of California, San Francisco (UCSF) Neurohospitalist Program and Fellowship, vice-chairman of the Department of Neurology, and the medical director of inpatient neurology. After graduating from Stanford University, Dr. Josephson earned a medical degree at Washington University in Saint Louis. He completed an internship in internal medicine and a residency in neurology at UCSF, where he was chief resident. He also completed fellowships in neurovascular neurology and behavioral neurology at UCSF. His current research focuses on systems and quality of inpatient neurologic care, including stroke, neurocritical care, and cognitive dysfunction. He is an associate professor of clinical neurology and holds the Carmen Castro Franceschi and Gladyne K. Mitchell Neurohospitalist Distinguished Professorship.

Kenneth W. Kizer, MD, MPH, is director of the Institute for Population Health Improvement of the University of California, Davis (UCD) Health System and Distinguished Professor in the UCD School of Medicine and Betty Irene Moore School of Nursing. He is one of very few persons elected to both the Institute of Medicine and the National Academy of Public Administration. Dr. Kizer's professional experience includes positions in academe and in the public and private sectors. He has been president, CEO, and chairman of the Medsphere Systems Corporation; founding president and CEO of the National Quality Forum; undersecretary for health in the US Department of Veterans Affairs and CEO of the nation's largest health care system; director of the California Department of Health Services; and director of the California Emergency Medical Services Authority. He has served on the US Preventive Services Task Force and as chairman of the Board of the California Wellness Foundation and on the governing boards of a number of managed-care and health information technology companies, foundations, professional associations, and nonprofit organizations. He has also served as an adviser to numerous foreign countries on health-related matters. Dr. Kizer is an honors graduate of Stanford University and the University of California, Los Angeles, and the recipient of two honorary doctorates. He is board certified in 6 medical specialties or subspecialties and he is the author of more than 400 articles, book chapters, and other reports. He is a fellow or distinguished fellow of 10 professional societies, a Fellow National of the international Explorer's Club, a founding member and past president of the international Wilderness Medical Society, and a former US Navy diver and diving medical officer.

**William C. Mann, PhD, OTRB,** is a Distinguished Professor and chair of occupational therapy, the director of the PhD Program in Rehabilitation Science, and the director of the Florida Institute on Disability and Rehabilitation (FIDR) of the University of Florida (UF). Within FIDR, Dr. Mann leads a Department of Defense–funded research initiative that is addressing issues related to rehabilitation of people who have combat injuries. He also serves as the director of the Rehabilitation Outcomes Research Center Research Enhancement Award Program of the North Florida/South Georgia Veterans Health System in Gainesville, Florida. Dr. Mann served as the principal investigator for the National Institute on Disability and Rehabilitation Research–funded Rehabilitation Engineering Research Center on Aging from 1991 to 2007; this work included a focus on uses of information technology in telehealth and home health and behavior monitoring. Before his appointment at UF, he was a professor at the University at Buffalo for 25 years. Dr. Mann is the author of more than 145 articles and book chapters on aging and independence and the author/editor of 5 books, and he was founder and from 1990 to 2000 coeditor of the journal *Technology and Disability*. He has served as the conference chair for the 1999, 2003, 2006, and 2008 International Conference on Aging, Disability and Independence and on the boards of the American Society on Aging and the Florida Council on Aging. His research and rehabilitation experience extends internationally to collaborations in Canada, Europe, Brazil, and Australia. Dr. Mann has more than 35 years of experience in rehabilitation and community-based programs, spanning research, service, and education, with a focus on applying technology to promote independence. Dr. Mann's current work addresses the needs of veterans who have disabilities, the application of home monitoring and communication technologies (telehealth and telerehabilitation), and tools for driver assessment and rehabilitation.

Linda J. Noble-Haeusslein, PhD, is a professor in the Department of Neurological Surgery and the Department of Physical Therapy and Rehabilitation Science of the University of California, San Francisco, holds the Alvera L. Kan Endowed Chair of Neurological Surgery, and is codirector and principal investigator of the Brain and Spinal Injury Center and codirector of the Neurobehavioral Core for Rehabilitation Research. Dr. Noble's research focuses on the neurobiology of traumatic injury to the central nervous system. In particular, her research uses experimental models of traumatic brain and spinal cord injury in the rodent to study the early events that contribute to cell injury and impair functional recovery. Her studies are funded by the National Institutes of Health and the Department of Defense. Dr. Noble received her BS from the University of Utah and her PhD from the University of California, Los Angeles. Dr. Noble is a member of numerous professional societies, including the Society for Neuroscience, the American Association of Anatomists, and the Society for Neurotrauma. She is on the editorial board of the *Journal of Neurotrauma* and the *International Journal of Neuroprotection and Neuroregeneration*. She has served on a previous Institute of Medicine committee that examined long-term outcomes of traumatic brain injury.

Edmond L. Paquette, MD, FACS, is a practicing urologist at Northern Virginia Urology PLLC, Fairfax, Virginia, and assistant professor of surgery at Virginia Commonwealth University School of Medicine, Inova Fairfax Campus, and assistant professor of surgery at the Uniformed Services University of the Health Sciences. He is a graduate of the University of Rhode Island and the Brown University School of Medicine. Dr. Paquette completed his general surgery internship at Madigan Army Medical Center in Ft. Lewis, Washington, and his urology residency at Walter Reed Army Medical Center. He served as the chief of the Urology Service at Womack Army Medical Center at Fort Bragg, North Carolina, until his honorable discharge from the US Army in June 2007. During his 13-year military career, Dr. Paquette also served in Germany, Bosnia, and Iraq. His research interests range from genitourinary war trauma to prostate cancer epidemiology. He has won numerous military awards, including the Iraqi Campaign Medal, Meritorious Service Medal, three Army Commendation Medals, Army Achievement Medal, National Defense Service Medal, Global War on Terror Service Medal, Armed Forces Service Medal, Army Service Ribbon, Overseas Ribbon, and NATO Medal. He is a diplomate of the American Board of Urology and a fellow of the American College of Surgeons. Additional professional memberships include the American Urological Association, the Society of Government Service Urologists, and the Society of Urologic Oncology.

**Alan L. Peterson, PhD, ABPP,** is a board-certified clinical health psychologist, professor, and chief of the Division of Behavioral Medicine in the Department of Psychiatry at the University of Texas Health Science Center at San Antonio. He also serves as the Deputy Chair for Military Collaborations and the director of the STRONG STAR Multidisciplinary PTSD Research Consortium. He completed a PhD in clinical psychology at Nova Southeastern University under the tutelage of Dr. Nathan Azrin, one of the founding fathers of behavior therapy. He completed a clinical psychology residency (internship) and postdoctoral fellowship in clinical health psychology at Wilford Hall Medical Center (WHMC). Dr. Peterson retired from the US Air Force in 2005 after 21 years of active duty service, including service as the chair of the Department of Psychology and the director of the Clinical Health Psychology Postdoctoral Fellowship Program at WHMC. While on active duty, he deployed in support of Operation Noble Eagle, Operation Enduring Freedom, and Operation Iraqi Freedom. Dr. Peterson has clinical and research experience in the areas of behavioral medicine, clinical health psychology, and combat-related stress disorders. He has conducted research in the areas of posttraumatic stress disorder, psychological risk, and resiliency, Tourette Syndrome, tobacco cessation, pain management, insomnia, weight management, and managing suicidal behaviors.

**Karol E. Watson, MD, PhD, FACC,** is a full-time cardiologist at the Geffen School of Medicine at the University of California, Los Angeles (UCLA). She is board certified in the fields of internal medicine and cardiology. Dr. Watson received her undergraduate degree from Stanford University, her medical degree from Harvard Medical School (magna cum laude), and her PhD in physiology from UCLA. She completed a residency in internal medicine and a fellowship in cardiology at UCLA, and continued there as part of the Specialty Training and Academic Research program and as Chief Fellow in Cardiovascular Diseases. Dr. Watson is director of the Women's Cardiovascular Center at UCLA, co-director of the UCLA Program in Preventative Cardiology, and director for the Center for Cholesterol and Hypertension Management. She is an associate professor of medicine in UCLA's Division of Cardiology and director of the UCLA Fellowship Program in Cardiovascular Diseases. She is a principal investigator for several large National Institutes of Health (NIH) studies, and serves on NIH Data, Safety, and Monitoring Boards and Steering Committees. She also currently serves as chairperson of the Clinical Chemistry and Clinical Toxicology Devices Panel of the Food and Drug Administration (FDA); she serves as a member of the National Cholesterol Education Program, a group responsible for updating the country's cholesterol management guidelines; she is a former vice president for the Association of Black Cardiologists; and is current chairperson of the Scientific Advisory Board for Womenheart, the national organization for women living with heart disease. The American Society of Hypertension recognizes Dr. Watson as a specialist in hypertension, she chairs the Cholesterol Committee of the Association of Black Cardiologists and serves on several NIH committees and panels, and is chair of the FDA Clinical Chemistry and Clinical Toxicology Devices Panel.